VIRUS

VIRUS

by Wolfhard Weidel

ANN ARBOR

THE UNIVERSITY OF MICHIGAN PRESS

Printed in the United States of America

Contents

VIRUS

1. *Introduction*

What is a virus?

Let us admit at the outset that we do not know; there is no brief and precise definition of the term. Perhaps the only practical definition would be: "Virus is what we are going to talk about in this book."

In the course of this guided tour through a living field of science the reader will come to understand why it is so difficult to give a completely accurate definition of the term virus. He will also realize, if his guide is successful, that we are on the very brink of a new and startling breakthrough in our knowledge about virus, and about life itself.

"Virus" is a Latin word meaning "poison." But as often happens in scientific language, the technical meaning of the term is both more specific and more complex than the simple translation would indicate. In the present case our knowledge is so incomplete that we must speak of virus not as a thing but as a concept. The haziness that surrounds the concept of virus is remarkably similar to the haziness that surrounds the concept of life. This similarity is not accidental. We shall soon see that nothing brings us so close to the riddle of life processes—

and to its solution—as viruses, whose strange behavior ties them intimately to occurrences in the smallest unit of life, the cell. For this reason we will spend a good deal of time considering cell processes. It is safe to predict that we shall really understand viruses only when the functions of the living cell hold no more mysteries for us, and vice versa. Until that time we must be content with a limited understanding, firmly based on experimental evidence, which clearly points out the direction in which further knowledge is to be sought. With this knowledge, however, we can ask concrete and purposeful questions.

Scientific method

Our job would be much simpler if we could observe viruses and cellular functions directly. But, just as the universe is too big for this, cells and viruses are too small. In such situations the scientist has to think of indirect methods for finding out what he wants to know. The principle of the indirect method is basically simple: what cannot be observed must be made to act upon what can be observed. The effects of this action are then measured and reveal the desired information.

In practice the indirect method is often a tedious business requiring much ingenuity and patience. In this book, however, we will deal mainly with direct answers to direct questions, intentionally ignoring all intervening technical complications. But remember that even such a simple matter as weighing an object becomes a problem when dealing with very small or very large objects. It would be impossible, for instance, to weigh on a scale a particle of matter that is not visible even under the strongest light-microscope. Scientists got around this difficulty—so that they can now weigh even virus particles—by measuring the particles' rate of sedimentation in a centrifuge. Since there is a logical and quantitative relationship between the sedimentation rate and the weight of the particle, the latter may be calculated from the former. This roundabout method is basically just as reliable as weighing with a scale. Of course the indirect method of weight determination—and other indirect methods as well—requires a great deal of apparatus. The grocer should consider himself lucky that he can do without an ultracentrifuge and still give his customers the correct weight. The scientist in the laboratory is no happier than the grocer would be with these complications; his apparatus is never an end in itself, as many laymen seem to think, but is often his only way to solve very simple problems.

Many people regard the laboratory with praiseworthy though quite unreasoning respect, shrugging the whole thing off with "That's beyond me." Thus a completely unnecessary barrier is erected between the elevated sphere where the scientist wanders and the ordinary everyday world. As a matter of fact, scientists always start with quite ordinary problems. What distinguishes the scientist is that he must be able to bring into quantitative relationship a number of perfectly simple thoughts and facts that do not seem to have even a qualitative relationship. Even in newly opened fields, a dense network of connected ideas can thus be formed very rapidly. No one who remembers the simple principles by which scientists arrive at these results needs to be frightened out of his wits by them.

The discovery of viruses

Viruses, as a matter of fact, were not really "discovered" in the same way that a previously unknown insect is discovered. Viruses first attracted notice through their effects. For decades no one saw a virus, although during this time scientists managed to find out quite a lot about them—even about their form.

The most obvious characteristic of viruses—the trait that gave them their name—is their "poisonous" effect on certain higher organisms, plants or animals, in which they cause disease. This in itself, of course, is nothing special; there are many substances that act as poisons. But viruses have one great peculiarity—no other poison increases in quantity when it is diluted. If a minute trace of sap is taken from a virus-diseased tobacco plant and rubbed on the leaf of a healthy plant, the latter will soon exhibit the same symptoms of tobacco mosaic disease (Fig. 1*b*). The sap of the second plant will then contain several million times more of the poison than it got from the first plant. With this sap several million more plants can be plunged into misfortune, their sap in turn can do away with more millions of plants, and so on ad infinitum.

The reader may raise an objection here. After all, this is no different from an infection due to harmful bacteria, which can be diluted through innumerable hosts because in each host they again multiply into hordes. This is a real objection, and for a time scientists thought that they were dealing with a form of bacteria.

One day, however, it occurred to someone to pass the disease-producing tobacco sap through a filter with pores so small that it was certain no real bacterium would be able to sneak through. And behold—the sap had lost none of its dangerous potency. What was one to think?

Beijerinck, the man who more than fifty years ago realized the importance of this experiment, felt certain that bacteria could not be the disease-producing agents in his sap filtrate. But he still did not dare go so far as to propose straightforwardly that a poisonous chemical substance, capable of reproducing itself, might be dissolved in his filtrate. He got himself out of the difficulty in a way that sounds peculiar but is still popular. He gave the thing a beautiful name—"contagium vivum fluidum" or "living fluid infectant"—and left it up to every man to think what he pleased about it. A diplomatic expression, if ever there was one! The fatal thing about such an evasion is that it tends to cut off questions that might lead to further experimentation, and instead opens the door to endless disputations which are as learned as they are fruitless.

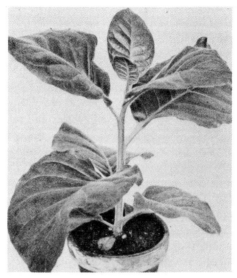

FIG. 1a. Healthy tobacco plant.

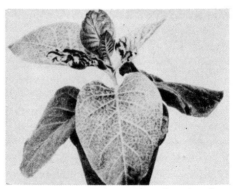

FIG. 1b. Tobacco plant infected with tobacco mosaic virus. (E. Bünning, *Lehrbuch der Pflanzenphysiologie.* Heidelberg, 1953.)

In this case, to be sure, the pitfall was avoided. Still, no immediate further progress was made—perhaps because shortly thereafter more examples were found of this contagious something that could not be trapped in a bacterial filter. Among these discoveries was the virus of the hoof-and-mouth disease, which was reported almost simultaneously with the tobacco mosaic virus. Scientists soon got used to such findings, and eventually the neutral name "virus" was agreed upon for filtrable disease-producing agents. The question whether a virus is living or nonliving did not even arise. Why shouldn't there be micro-organisms even smaller than bacteria? And so, for a long time, viruses remained under the guardianship of the bacteriologists, who did not particularly love them because viruses would not learn to grow on artificial media (only in living organisms, or at least in cell tissues, will viruses reproduce themselves). This fact, unpleasant enough for the research worker, was made a further criterion for calling a given disease-producing agent a virus.

Sensation

Not until about twenty years ago, when the chemist Stanley made a discovery which seemed to contradict the concept of viruses as living organisms, was there any real cause for excitement. Stanley had once again taken up the infectious tobacco sap and isolated some crystals from it, which appeared to be the tobacco mosaic virus (Fig. 2). A minute quantity of these crystals dissolved in water proved to be just as infectious for healthy tobacco plants as the fresh sap of a plant already ailing from the mosaic disease.

It seemed as if the causal agent for tobacco mosaic virus disease was really just a lifeless chemical substance, crystallizable like cooking salt, yet capable of multiplying like an organism in the tobacco plant, to the latter's harm. There may have been philosophical qualms, but for the

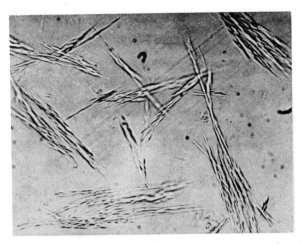

FIG. 2. Crystalline needles of tobacco mosaic virus, enlarged approximately 500 times. Each needle consists of many thousands of rod-shaped virus particles, which are not visible at this low magnification. (G. Schramm, *Die Biochemie der Viren.* Heidelberg, 1954.)

moment there were few doubters, especially because it soon became possible to obtain further virus types in crystalline form. The most important immediate effect of the sensational "living crystals" was that now more and more chemists and physicists began to take an interest in viruses. To their minds the fact that entities formerly considered as micro-organisms had suddenly turned out to be crystallizable substances opened up a whole new field of activity.

Crystals are made up of large numbers of smaller particles, arranged in regular order. In a virus crystal these smaller particles are all practically identical, and each of them represents a virus "molecule" (Fig. 3). Each molecule, in turn, is composed of an enormous number of various atoms (carbon, hydrogen, nitrogen, and others). The atoms in a molecule adhere much more strongly to each other than do the molecules in the

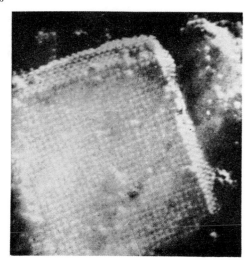

FIG. 3. A rectangular crystal of tobacco necrosis virus seen under the electron microscope. At this enormous enlargement (approximately 50,000 times) one can distinguish the individual (in this case spherical) virus particles, which have aggregated to form the crystal. (R. Markham, K. M. Smith, and R. W. G. Wyckoff. *Nature,* 161 [1948], 760.)

crystal. Therefore the atoms do not separate when the crystal is dissolved in water, but the molecules, as units, become independent, each going its own way.

The very first experiments with virus crystals indicated that a single virus molecule, once it gets into a suitable organism, can set off an avalanche of reproduction of itself, and give rise to millions more of such molecules. This raised the question whether the ability for self-reproduction could somehow be explained from the fine structure of the virus molecule. This question seemed doubly important because there are certain components of every living cell which were also thought to be capable of self-reproduction. These special cell-components are the inheritance factors, called "genes." One imagined the genes as self-reproducing giant molecules. No one had ever obtained genes in purified form, however, and therefore the discovery that viruses can be crystallized was particularly welcome. Now, at last, one type of "self-replicating" giant molecule, purified of all contaminants, was available and it became possible to move in on this with the whole arsenal of laboratory methods: to study its construction, and, possibly, to follow it into the living organism to examine its effects. The reason why the mechanism of reproduction is of such particular interest will become clear as we explore the subject further. We will see that it is the key to an understanding not only of virus but also of life processes in general.

II. *Reproduction*

Mechanism versus essence

Perhaps some readers will take unkindly to the word "mechanism" as applied to vital processes. Haven't we long surpassed primitive mechanistic conceptions, especially in relation to the phenomenon of life? There is no answer to this except a counterquestion: What justification is there for the popular but superficial belief that "mechanistic" and "primitive" go together?

Any run-of-the-mill philosopher who considers himself miles above mechanistic ideas can collect an audience and hold forth about God and the World. But there is reason to suspect him of earning his applause mostly by simplifying things. The true scientist, on the other hand, has difficulty in explaining his thoughts just because he must insist on a thorough understanding of more or less complicated mechanisms. He can consider something to be explained and understood only if it can be traced back to an interaction of tangible factors—a mechanism. To understand such a mechanism at all it is necessary to understand it completely, so that a certain minimum of intellectual effort is required even if one only wants to rethink it. Where a mechanism is concerned, it is useless to "interpret its essence." An incompetent auto mechanic gives himself away by "explaining" unfixed car troubles with a flow of words, but it is only the naïve who will be taken in by such pseudo explanations.

Of course, none of the natural sciences deals exclusively with screw-and-lever types of mechanisms. Chemical, electrical, selectional, sometimes purely mathematical mechanisms, to mention just a few, may be involved. A mathematical mechanism, for example, is expressed by the logical structure of a certain formula describing correctly the behavior of atoms, which could not be made evident by means of a model.

In concluding this little sermon on the mechanistic principles of the natural sciences, we might ask again: Is it really "primitive" for generations of laboratory workers painstakingly to add observation to observation in order, at last, to deduce the basic mechanism which in turn explains each individual observation? It certainly seems to me that this manner of arriving at knowledge about our world shows more respect for the wonderful organization of the microcosm and macrocosm than any "philosophical" interpretation based on a few general experiences, no matter how deep such an interpretation may seem.

Two reproductive schemes

Since a discussion of mechanisms cannot be avoided, let us jump right in and ask about the most important characteristics of living cells and the mechanisms responsible for them. We will concentrate on vital processes in individual cells, because virus reproduction takes place inside the cell and nowhere else.

Let us have a look at the bacterial cell. In a suitable environment it multiplies rapidly (often, alas, to our misfortune). First it increases in mass, then divides into two daughter cells; each of these then repeats the same process, until 2, 4, 8, 16, 32, and finally billions of cells have arisen from the original one. Thus in every generation (or in equivalent units of time) the number of cells is doubled. This manner of reproduction is called "geometric."

A totally different manner of reproduction applies, for example, to the workers of a bee colony. Here the queen lays only one egg at a time; from this egg emerges only one worker bee, who, for her part, cannot lay an egg. Therefore the number of workers in the colony increases by the same amount in the same interval, and such a manner of reproduction is called "arithmetic." Let us remember these two types of reproduction because they will be important later.

We now know two possible schemes of reproduction, but this doesn't tell us anything about the operative force behind them. Should we accept the pseudo explanation that it is the "life force" which is involved? A student of economics might as well believe that the rate of interest is the force which increases a bank account!

We know, of course, that interest is earned only through work performed somewhere—through conversion of energy and goods. The same is true for the "interest," in the form of billions of daughter cells, earned from a multiplying bacterial cell. Incidentally, the daughter cells are constantly added to the "capital," causing the accumulation of compound interest, which is just another way of saying the increase is geometric. Anyway, the operative force is to be sought in the transfer of energy and material, and we have to investigate how these two function in the cell.

Assembly-line reproduction

Many transformations which cells can perform have long been known—for example, the fermentation of sugar into alcohol and carbon dioxide performed by yeast cells. Pasteur, who discovered this process, considered alcoholic fermentation to be a "life function" of the yeast cell. Though a master of neat experiment and shrewd conclusion, he oddly enough contented himself here with this pseudo explanation without feeling the need for further experiments. In this way, to be sure, he accommodated the habits of thinking, or feeling, of his contemporaries. For that reason a very simple experiment, which was performed two years after his death, caused a stir quite out of keeping with the scientific ingenuity involved. It was simply found that it is possible to ferment sugar into alcohol and carbon dioxide with a cell-free extract made from yeast.

You will remember that the discovery of the crystallizability of tobacco mosaic virus caused a similar sensation. Excitement is aroused when preconceived notions, which are firmly anchored in the public mind, are knocked over by facts. We may expect quite a few more such sensations when other preconceived notions are undermined.

The sugar-fermenting yeast extract proved to be the stimulus for more and more successful penetration into the chemical mechanisms of living cells. Later on viruses provided a further impetus in the same direction. Since the yeast extract was capable of transforming a well-known chemical substance, namely sugar, into other equally well-known chemical substances, namely alcohol and carbon dioxide, it had to be assumed that there was something in it which effected this transformation. The mysterious "life force" was luckily (otherwise one might not have bothered to investigate further) out of the question here, even for its most ardent adherents. To assume that this "life force" was still roaming about in a fluid which otherwise gave no signs of life would no doubt have lowered it too much in the eyes of its defenders. Further knowledge could now be expected only from those seeking concrete mechanisms in living things. According to mechanistic conceptions the yeast extract, and thus also the living yeast cells from which it came, must contain substances which somehow chemically react with sugar and cause it to split up. The job now was to isolate these substances, or "enzymes" as they are called, from the extract in order to study them more closely.

The problem turned out to be far more difficult than it was at first assumed, and it was finally solved only a few years ago. There were two reasons for this: First, the enzymes sought were very sensitive, so to begin with special methods had to be developed in order not to destroy or inactivate them during the purification attempts. The development of a more delicate experimental technique was very time-consuming. Secondly, however, it turned out that an unexpectedly large number of enzymes and subsidiary substances, differing quite thoroughly in their chemical construction and especially in their chemical effect, were present in the yeast extract. and that all these had to work together if sugar was to be split into alcohol and carbon dioxide. This transformation does not, as was first thought, take place in one jump, but only step by step, over many intermediate chemical stages which the sugar must pass through until the two end products finally emerge. Each intermediate transformation requires a specific enzyme, just as every manipulation in the construction of an automobile on an assembly line requires a specific worker. If one worker is missing, and cannot be replaced, then, in this production system, no automobiles emerge from the factory.

A detailed reconstruction of the chemical assembly line, which, in the yeast extract or cell, works on the sugar, took tremendous care and skill. This is not surprising considering that about a dozen different enzymes take part in the job. Today, however, it is possible to isolate all of these enzymes in pure form, put them into separate bottles, and keep them on the shelf. If they are mixed together again, and sugar solution is added, its transformation into alcohol and carbon dioxide begins immediately.

An assembly line is really a very apt model for the chemical happenings when the cell breaks down substances it takes in from the outside, shapes them into derivatives, or uses them as building blocks for the construction of entirely different material. It is now known, due to innumerable experimental studies, that these transformations always take place step by step. The "conveyor belts" are already "mounted" in the cells complete with "workers" in the form of the most varied types of enzyme molecules, each of which performs a particular task—only that task, and no other. The performance of the task does not permanently change the enzyme molecule. One could imagine that the enzyme might be transformed into something else itself by effecting the chemical transformation of another substance which is floating along in the cell fluid, and to which it is adapted. This, in fact, does happen momentarily, but when the reaction is completed in a split-second, only one of the two partners is transformed. The other, the enzyme particle, emerges completely unaffected, like the phoenix from the ashes, and can immediately repeat the same process. Of course a human worker is not built into the auto, nor is he harmed in the performance of his task on the assembly line—at least not if he is careful. Otherwise this would be an expensive and impractical business which neither the Ford Motor Company nor the cell could afford.

In other words each enzyme works as a so-called catalyst for a specific chemical transformation which could not happen without it; the enzyme enables the transformation to take place without itself being permanently involved in it. The chemical industry also uses catalysts, for instance in the production of nitrogenous fertilizer from the atmosphere, or for the transformation of coal into gasoline, though these catalysts are chem ically very different from enzymes.

Now we know how substances, taken up from the environment, are transformed by the cell. The reasons for these chemical exertions are usually obvious: growth and reproduction require the formation of additional amounts of all the enzymes and other materials of which the cell itself consists. Since practically none of the necessities are found ready-made among the chemical substances of the environment, the cell has only one option: it must construct the material of which it, itself, consists from those chemical substances in the environ- ment which it is able to transform and reshape on its chemical assembly lines. Such substances are "nutrients" for the cell. The cells of micro-organisms are especially skilled here: from a water solution with only a few salts and some simple carbon source such as glycerin they are able to construct the most complicated chemical molecules for the maintenance and increase of their own kind.

Making energy

But what about those cases where the cell seems to use elaborate assembly lines to make a product which is useless and is therefore eventually eliminated? For example the yeast cell which, with its production of alcohol, provided the first glimpse into the chemical methods of living organisms, cannot do a thing with the alcohol it has made. Why then does it go to all the trouble? Merely to get drunk on the product of its private moonshine industry? Well, that does happen on occasion, and so thoroughly that the cell usually doesn't survive the hangover. Such intoxication, however, is ac- cidental and can hardly be the main purpose for the enormous effort required to make alcohol. Something much more remarkable is involved.

Before we go on, we have to consider first what is

required, in addition to bricks, mortar, and beams, if one wants to build a house. From what we have said earlier, the reader will be able to guess: work must be performed, and for that supplies of energy are needed (sandwiches for the workers, electricity or gasoline for cement-mixers, cranes, etc.). The cell is in the same position when it wants to expand its house (with which it is identical), that is, when it wants to grow and multiply. This cannot be accomplished either without work, for which the cell must have a source of energy.

Being an ingenious chemist, the cell naturally turns to chemical sources of energy, which it taps by means of special assembly lines, whose apparent end products are then useless for the cell (for example, alcohol and carbon dioxide for the yeast cell). This type of assembly line, unlike the synthesizing type, is not geared for a chemical end product; rather, it is a "disassembly" line, which means that a given chemical substance, for example sugar, is decomposed along this path by means of chemical transformations in order to yield energy, a "physical" product.

The fact that chemical transformations can produce energy is so well known that it is hardly necessary to say more about it. In daily life the chemical transformation most frequently employed to produce energy is combustion. Combustion is a process by which atmospheric oxygen reacts with a combustible substance to produce heat (though not necessarily fire). Living cells also frequently make use of this method because, of all energy-producing chemical processes available to them, this one, here called "respiration," produces the most energy. However, many cell types possess remarkable special assembly lines for producing energy even when oxygen is not available. We have already discussed one of these special mechanisms: alcoholic fermentation. It is a fact that the cell makes use of this rather uneconomical means of producing energy only when atmospheric oxygen is unavailable. When oxygen is available, the assembly line for fermentation is automatically shut off and replaced by another using atmospheric oxygen to transform sugar not into carbon dioxide and alcohol (which is combustible and thus still contains considerable quantities of unused energy) but into carbon dioxide and water. From these two end products no more energy is to be derived by chemical means.

Utilizing energy

How does the cell utilize the energy which it derives from the decomposition of nutrients? For a long time this was thought to be very simple: where chemical transformations produce energy, this energy usually appears in the form of heat. It was therefore supposed that the cell is interested in heat, just as we are when we burn coal under a steam kettle. But as a matter of fact, there isn't much the cell can do with heat energy for the following reason.

Energy is used in the cell wherever complex chemical structures are to be built up from simple building blocks. Such building-block molecules, however, are not obliging enough to co-operate if they are only warmed up a little. But they will if they are charged with energy in a way transforming them into stretched springs, so to speak, which, when released by the slightest push, tend to snap and intermesh quite easily. How is this charging with energy to be accomplished? First, take a "special molecule" which is particularly rich in energy (we will find out in a minute where it comes from) and let it snap a little, but not completely—just enough to unite it with the building-block molecule which is to be charged. Some of the energy brought into the union by the "special molecule" will be left over in the complex formed; this remaining energy is enough to cause a second "snapping" during which the real purpose is accomplished—a final meshing of the charged building-block molecule with another one which need not even be charged. The remainder of the "special molecule," whose energy is now completely spent, then extricates itself from the complex once the two building-block molecules are firmly joined. Through the use of one after another of these charged "special molecules" as sources of energy, simple building-block molecules, consisting of a few atoms, can be joined together to form chains of any length, nets, and complex spatial structures—the so-called giant molecules.

Such giant molecules are very important in the cell structure. Together with complexes of an even higher order, they make up the major cell apparatus. The enzyme molecules, with which we have already made acquaintance, belong in this company. Some of these enzymes, in turn, play an important part as skilled assembly-line workers in the "snapping" process just described; they see to it that everything runs smoothly and leads to the desired products by allowing only the proper building-block molecules to come together.

Of course we haven't reached the end of the story. Where does the cell get its enormous requirements of "special molecules"? They arise as the products of the energy assembly lines (respiration and fermentation) which thus convert sugar not only into carbon dioxide and water (or alcohol) but also into the chemically charged springs. Energy, which is released during the decomposition of sugar, is built into special molecules and stored, instead of being allowed to escape practically uselessly as heat. The charged molecules are immediately utilized in the active cell, but after performance of their tasks, their discharged remainders return to the respiratory and fermenting assembly lines to be recharged again and again into the energy-rich form. The shift from charged to discharged state and back again is very rapid and therefore the absolute quantity per cell of this remarkable molecule is very small. For this reason, too, in spite of their important role as middlemen they long remained undiscovered.

From a chemical point of view the processes we have been discussing are perfectly straightforward. Nowadays it is even possible to induce considerable portions of this chemical orchestra to keep in tune in the test tube instead of the cell and to produce various materials on demand. Crude matter, so often despised by dogmatic philosophers, can certainly accomplish a lot more quite on its own than their kind would have deemed possible —or shall we say, would have been able to find out.

Division of labor

Now, let us try to think the chemical interactions in the cell through to the end. Yet is there really an end? Growing and multiplying cells obviously synthesize more and more of all the chemical constituents of which each of them is composed. Of course the cell components must always be made in the appropriate sorts, amounts and proportions, otherwise yeast, typhus, or any other kinds of cells would soon become nonfunctioning monsters. We note, however, that a yeast cell always produces yeast cells, a typhus cell more typhus cells, and so forth.

The material for this synthesis is derived from the environment, since even a cell cannot make something from nothing. Usually one and the same nutrient, for instance sugar (or glycerin, or acetic acid), serves for the production of both energy and cell material, depending on whether it is worked on by a decomposing (energy-deriving) or a synthesizing assembly line. This, of course, means an important simplification of the system, as does the fact that energy, no matter from what source it is derived, is always stored in the same types of "special molecules." The assembly lines of each cell are so interlocked by means of branches and cross connections that the result is an all-encompassing dy-

namic network of chemical reactions constantly operating
in all directions.

Alone, however, this dynamic network is not enough
to give life to the cell. The chemical reaction-chains or
assembly lines within the cell must obviously be so
attuned to each other that in the end they produce just
those chemo-technical apparatuses which together *are*
"the cell"! The production goes around in a circle, and
thus becomes completely its own purpose. For example,
the cell needs enzymes of various types with which to
mediate chemical reaction-chains—and conversely, it
needs the reaction-chains in order to produce, among
other things, new enzyme molecules to replace those
which are ready to retire or have been accidentally damaged, or, when a daughter cell is to be produced, to
duplicate the whole inventory. In the last analysis the
enzyme molecules assure their own reproduction, but
obviously very indirectly, because their entire activity in
the cell consists in the performance of some single
manipulation on one assembly line. By doing its duty in
its own place and making sure that "its" assembly line
runs smoothly, each enzyme molecule contributes
toward the proper functioning of the entire factory,
represented by the network of chemical interactions. In
this way, and only in this way—and at quite another
point in the reaction network—more of such enzyme
molecules can be produced.

This extremely indirect reproductive mechanism, which
is possible only with a very highly organized division of
labor at interlocking assembly lines, must also undoubtedly apply to the remaining cell components. They
are all dependent on one another for their reproduction,
or enlargement in the growing cell, or their regeneration
in the event of wear.

At this point we ought to have some inkling of what
is meant by the simple statement: "The cell reproduces
itself." This "itself" may perhaps apply to the whole cell,

to express the autonomy of the integrated process as seen from the outside. If one delves deeper, however, and looks at the reproduction of the individual cell components, one finds that these do not reproduce autonomously, but in the most indirect manner imaginable. Yet for certain cell components there may be limitations to the strictness of the principle of indirect reproduction. This we will have to discuss later on.

Dead or alive

Now at last we can begin to understand what is meant by "Life" on the level of the autonomous cell. A chemical reaction-network, which, by running its production around in a circle, maintains and reproduces itself, is a living thing, and a living cell is such a reaction-network. If the dynamic of such a network is even temporarily halted, as by freezing the whole system, then obviously at that very moment only an accumulation of various materials remains, which together are just as "dead" as each individual component was "dead" —before and after the stoppage! The terms "living matter" or "live matter" are based on grave misunderstandings, as we can see now. If one just prevents the production of the network from going around in a circle, without, however, blocking the dynamic, then a considerable part of the chemical reactions may continue to function for a while; nevertheless in the end the network is condemned to "death" because it is no longer capable of completely regenerating itself. This is also the normal cause of death in higher organisms. They must delegate special tasks to many of their cells, which these latter can only perform by sacrificing the productive self-sufficiency of their networks. Thereby they are condemned. Sooner or later the sentence is carried out and the whole organism must perish. A normal death in this sense does not exist among unicellular organisms. They are exclusively subject to accidents. In principle they live forever—or else they couldn't live at all.

Biochemists have not yet been able to reconstruct a living organism in the test tube; no matter how many enzymes, and other materials isolated from the cell, were ingeniously assembled, the result was only a part of a cell's artificial reaction-network. The reason for this is not that the components of the mixture behave somehow differently in the test tube than in the cell; rather, no way has yet been found to reconstruct chemical reaction-networks which would synthesize *all* their component parts, the only way of making the whole assembly capable of regeneration and reproduction. For the biochemist it might eventually prove impossible to achieve this end for mere technical reasons. At present he also still lacks important insights into details of the real structure of self-contained reaction-networks, particularly with respect to the point at which the whole thing "bites its tail." Only the principles involved are so far beginning to emerge.

Viruses as bloodhounds

Here, at last, we come to viruses again. Viruses reproduce "themselves" exclusively within living cells. Closer investigation has shown that here, too, "reproduce themselves" is not to be read as completely autonomous virus reproduction. Rather the situation is the following: A virus particle temporarily takes over a specific role in the reaction-network of the cell it has infected, with the result that this network is redirected and now produces large quantities of virus particles instead of normal cell components. Viruses, in other words, are no more "alive" than enzyme molecules or any other normal cell components; they also accomplish their reproduction in a very indirect manner, specifically by means of the preconstructed reaction-network of the host cell.

The peculiar adaptability of the virus into the host cell apparatus must obviously be connected with the chemical structure of viruses, which is so similar to that of certain normal cell components as to allow the virus to take the place of the latter. This place is apparently located at a point in the reaction-network which is of crucial importance for the completion of the cycle; it is the place normally held by the material carriers of heredity of the cell, the genetic factors or genes.

Later we will go into the detailed reasons for this assumption, which, by the way, is why the theoretical sciences are so interested in viruses. First we must learn how viruses may be handled so that they can be used to probe previously inaccessible centers of activity in the reaction-network of living cells.

III. *The Virus in the Laboratory*

Hunting for viruses

Microbe-hunting has been a popular sport since the days of Leeuwenhoek, and today unicellular organisms are still being discovered with the use of a microscope. If viruses are the quarry, however, not even an electron microscope will be of any use, although virus particles can, in fact, be seen with one. Actually looking at a new virus is always the last step in its description and discovery. A highly concentrated and purified preparation must already be available for observation through the electron microscope; otherwise it is impossible to distinguish the virus from the many tiny structures which appear on the electron microscope screen regardless of what is being looked at. To find a single bacterium in a small soil sample with an ordinary microscope would be difficult; finding a virus particle with an electron microscope would be more hopeless than looking for the proverbial needle in the haystack. The electron-microscopic haystack is due to the enormous enlargement which is necessary if the virus particle is to be seen at all. A crumb of a millimeter in diameter would be a sixty-yard monster at this magnification, but most virus particles would barely look as large as a pinhead.

An additional difficulty is that an unknown virus type can be of any shape. Cells generally have some characteristics in common, and, in spite of great variability, a cell can usually be recognized as such. Viruses, on the other hand, have no typical form; some types are spherical, others angular, still others are rod- or needle-shaped, and some look like little tadpoles or clubs.

How are viruses ever discovered if they cannot be seen, even under the electron microscope, until they are already concentrated and purified? The answer was given in the first chapter of this book: Viruses are recognized by their effects on living organisms. To do experiments with viruses means to work with these effects; experiments must be so designed that under the same conditions, the same effect is always produced in the same way and thus becomes reproducible. Once this has been accomplished it becomes possible to measure virus quantities, the most important basis for further scientific work.

An indirect method for measuring amounts of a substance through its effect is called a "quantitative test." It is especially useful to the biochemist in separating some substance that interests him from inactive impurities. The unknown substance may be a hormone, vitamin, or virus; without a dependable quantitative test, which represents his "eye," the biochemist is helpless and wouldn't even think of attempting the isolation.

Before designing a virus test, one must, of course, be certain that the effects observed on plants or animals are really due to a virus. Among plants, for example, there are occasionally diseases caused by mineral deficiencies in the soil which can be mistaken for virus infections. The disease in question must be transferable to healthy plants, which is sometimes difficult to prove because viruses may require special conditions for transfer.

In the case of animals and man it is usually not too

difficult to show that a given disease-producing agent is transferable. This alone, however, doesn't prove that it is a virus; it could be a bacterium or fungus which is hard to grow on an artificial medium. Even if the causal agent passes through a bacterial filter, we cannot be absolutely sure it is a virus; some types of viruses are adsorbed or even inactivated by such filters and thus do not show up in the filtrate. On the other hand, certain micro-organisms, which are certainly not viruses, are nevertheless small enough to slip through the pores of such a filter. Size, in other words, is not an absolute criterion for distinguishing viruses from genuine micro-organisms, although it can be used in conjunction with other characteristics.

Nowadays, anyway, the problem of proving that a certain disease is caused by a virus doesn't come up very often. The most important virus diseases have long been known, and the tedious search for new ones seems rather less appealing than collecting butterflies. Basic research is usually concerned with delving more deeply into experimental material already at hand. Still, the collection and typing of pathogens is essential for the control of epidemics and sometimes, in the course of this work, incidental discoveries are made which turn out to be invaluable for the solution of basic problems. Among viruses the outstanding example of this sort was the discovery of a virus type which infects bacteria only. This will be the major subject of our discourses later on.

Growing viruses in the laboratory

A zoologist specializing in spiders can probably get along without growing them in his laboratory. Whenever necessary, he can go out and collect a few spiders, or just observe them in their natural habitat. Not so the virologist; he must find a way of growing his specimens in or near his laboratory, or else all further work on them would be impossible. Naturally his aim will be to get as large a yield of viruses as possible in a way which is technically as simple as possible. Some virus types are more difficult to cultivate than others; for example, until recently, it was very difficult to culture the poliomyelitis virus.

Of course for purposes of basic research one would always pick a virus which is easy to grow and purify so that this part of the work can be routinely carried out by a laboratory assistant. It does not matter whether the virus chosen from this point of view is also of great practical importance. Information derived from work with one virus type can usually be applied to other types of viruses.

If viruses were self-reproducing organisms in the true sense, like bacterial cells, there would be no difficulty in growing them on artificial media. It usually doesn't take long to find a suitable combination of nutrients for a bacterial culture. However, as we already know, a virus particle cannot use the most lovingly concocted specialities of the media-kitchen; the virus particle can only multiply by entering a preformed network of bio-chemical assembly lines, and these can as yet be found only in living cells. Consequently the first step in growing viruses is to grow living cells, which can be infected with the virus and thereby made to produce more virus.

Sometimes, as in the case of tobacco mosaic virus (TMV), this is no problem. Tobacco seeds are sown and allowed to grow up into magnificent leafy plants to furnish all the living cells needed for infecting with viruses. Under suitable conditions a local infection spreads through the whole plant and soon practically every plant cell will be producing quantities of new viruses. A small tobacco plot yields a large supply of TMV which can be extracted from the plants, purified, and used for further experiments.

It is too bad that not all types of virus will grow in tobacco plants or other organisms which are equally plentiful. Unfortunately, most viruses have a rather small range of possible hosts. This means that each type of virus can only multiply in one or at most a few organisms. In most cases not even the whole organism but only the cells of certain tissues are involved in virus reproduction. Culturing viruses may thus be a wasteful business if the whole plant or animal has to be grown and then only part of it can be used; in addition there is the problem of separating the virus-containing tissues from the rest. It becomes expensive, too, when the host animals required are monkeys as for the polio virus, or cattle for the virus of hoof-and-mouth disease.

One way out, in such cases, is not to grow the whole animals but only those of their tissues which can be used for virus production. Tissue culture is an art which has been practiced for some decades. Liver, kidney, nerve, or connective tissues can be grown in bottles of nutrient solution kept at body temperature in the incubator. This art has nowadays found broadest application in virus research, for purely scientific purposes as well as for practical ones. For example, large quantities of polio virus are produced now by infecting the kidney tissues of monkeys. The resulting yield is then used to make the polio vaccine which was headline news only recently. It is, of course, difficult to produce a vaccine which is both effective and harmless from the active virus, and this accounts for some of the early failures (see Chapter VII).

Tissue culture, though a useful technique, is not ideal for research purposes because keeping the tissues going is very time-consuming. Cells of higher organisms are extremely sensitive; they must frequently be transplanted to fresh nutrient media and, in spite of every care, there is always the danger of bacterial attack which can destroy a whole culture in no time because the attackers are much more robust than the tissue cells. Keeping up a fresh supply of cultures is thus a considerable technical problem. A constant supply of fresh cultures is absolutely necessary, however, because the virus-infected cells do not continue to produce viruses indefinitely but soon disintegrate. This self-destruction of the virus-infected cell is nearly inevitable and later on we will study the reason for it.

A creative new look at the problem of virus culture resulted in an improvement of technique which removed some of the difficulties. It was found that quite a number of viruses which are pathogenic for animals and humans can be grown in the cells of a chicken embryo in the egg. Here too the whole chicken is not needed. In fact the tissues in question are not part of the finished chicken; they just enclose the developing embryo like a sack. This sack, called the chorioallantoic membrane, is like a lining for the inside of the eggshell (Fig. 4). An egg, containing a partially developed chicken embryo, is carefully opened at the blunt end; the embryo is removed and a virus solution is introduced into the cavity. The cells of the lining will be infected by the virus; they will produce quantities of new virus and release it back into the liquid (Fig. 5). Here the tissue culture is automatically sterile until it is actually used for virus production, at which point it no longer matters because the lining cells will have finished making viruses in a

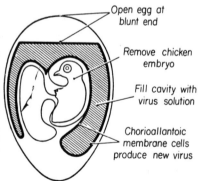

FIG. 4. Diagram of longitudinal section of an egg with partially developed chicken embryo. Virus solution is introduced into the cavity indicated by shading. (After W. I. B. Beveridge and F. M. Burnet, *The Cultivation of Viruses and Rickettsiae in the Chick Embryo.* London, 1946, 1953.)

Open egg at blunt end

Remove chicken embryo

Fill cavity with virus solution

Chorioallantoic membrane cells produce new virus

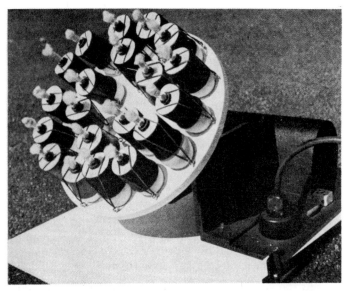

FIG. 5. A battery of de-embryonated chicken eggs ready for virus production. The opened ends are covered by rubber caps. Glass tubes with cotton plugs permit air to enter and facilitate introduction or removal of fluids. The eggs are mounted on a wooden disk which rotates slowly at an angle. The whole setup is kept in the incubator. (M. Sprössig, Jena.)

few hours. A few stray bacteria would not be able to grow into menacing numbers in such a short time; even a possible major contamination caused by sloppy technique in opening the egg can be counteracted by adding a bit of penicillin, streptomycin, or other antibiotic to the culture solution. This will prevent the multiplication of any bacteria without affecting the reproduction of the virus.

Could anything be simpler? It is hard to believe, but the answer is "yes," and here we come back to the virus which specializes in attacking bacteria. The technical name for these bacterial viruses is bacteriophage (literally "bacteria eaters") or phage, for short. The work with phage has led to more important discoveries than all other virus work taken together. And growing phage is no problem at all: a simple nutrient broth is infected with suitable bacteria. In a few hours the previously clear fluid will look turbid because it now contains millions of bacterial cells. A few drops of phage solution are added, and after an interval the solution again clears. If all has gone well, each cubic centimeter should now contain up to a billion new phage particles but practically no more whole, live bacteria. This is a large yield with a small amount of effort. A single hard-working experimenter using the egg method may have to spend up to $2,000 a year for eggs, whereas one using phage can do with less than a tenth of that amount for the same purpose.

Measuring quantities

At the beginning of this chapter we said that in order to concentrate and purify a virus a quantitative test is needed making it possible to measure virus quantities at least in a comparative way. A method permitting a direct count of virus particles would be even better, of course, because thereby one would measure absolute instead of relative amounts of virus. Furthermore, as will be seen, many experiments digging deeper into the mysteries of virus reproduction depend entirely on an absolute method whereby single virus particles can be counted.

The most universally applicable comparative method of estimating virus quantities is the following: A "standard preparation" of the virus in question is made up to a concentration where it causes the expected effect, usually disease or death, in only about half of the host organisms to which it is applied, and not in the other half. Experience has shown that such a balance of effect between 50 per cent positive and 50 per cent negative is quite readily reproducible, and, for obvious statistical reasons, the more so the larger the number of experimental objects.

By testing a solution containing an unknown amount of virus in the same way, it can be compared with the standard preparation. If, for example, the unknown solution must be diluted five times before not more than 50 per cent of the experimental organisms sicken or die, then it obviously contains five times as much virus per unit volume as the standard. This comparative method is useful for following the increase of virus quantities during purification procedures, or, on the other hand, the inactivation of viruses during experiments to combat virus disease.

Since the absolute quantity of virus in the standard preparation remains unknown, nothing can be said about absolute quantities in the solutions compared to it. Until recently there was no way at all to determine absolute virus quantities. For plant viruses there still is none; for some animal viruses such measuring techniques which were first worked out with phage have now been adapted.

A simple and obvious example of the statistical test involves viruses which multiply within a chicken embryo and kill it in the process. The procedure is to inject some test solution into a number of partially developed eggs—this time without removing the embryo—and then to wait and see what percentage of the embryos die.

A quicker comparative test is based on the ability of certain animal-pathogenic viruses to cause red blood cells to form clumps (agglutination), which can be seen with the naked eye. Agglutination needs a certain minimum level of virus concentration to occur. Virus solutions of unknown concentration just have to be diluted to this level to be compared with one another. The solution which had to be diluted most must have contained the most virus. The dilution factor in each case, called the "agglutination titer," is a relative measure of virus quantity.

Finally there are certain serological tricks for comparing virus quantities. They are similar to the well-known Wassermann reaction for syphilis, but we need not go into details. Quantitative tests for plant viruses are especially tedious, for one single test often requires the use of a large number of plants. A pleasant exception is made by tobacco mosaic virus which on a certain strain of tobacco plants produces no systemic infection of the whole host. Instead, when the leaves of this plant are painted with a TMV solution, the infection remains limited to single spots on the leaf which soon become discolored and are easily seen (Fig. 6). In each of these

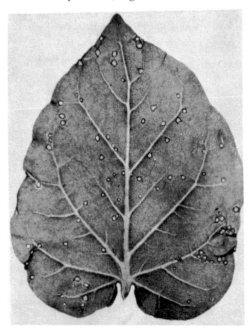

FIG. 6. Single infections of TMV on a leaf of *Nicotiana glutinosa*. (G. Schramm.)

"local lesions" the virus has settled into a relatively small group of cells which reproduced it and died, but the infection has not spread. Within certain limits of concentration, the nunber of these local lesions will be approximately proportional to the virus concentration; in other words, a doubly concentrated solution would produce twice as many spots.

One might think that here at least is a method for counting individual virus particles. It is true that each spot most probably does derive from a single particle entering a leaf cell which was slightly scratched when the virus solution was applied. Unfortunately, however, there isn't always a damaged—and consequently receptive—leaf cell wherever a virus particle happens to land. Thus a certain incalculable part of the applied virus is wasted on unreceptive cells, and in the same way receptive cells are wasted because no virus particle happens to come in contact with them. In fact this whole test, which at first seemed so cheeringly straightforward, begins to look rather dubious. Nevertheless it is possible to get fairly dependable results with some modifications of the method. For instance, one half of each leaf can be painted with the virus solution of unknown concentration, and a standard solution applied to the other half. The two halves of as many leaves as possible are then compared as to number of lesions. The more diligent the experimenter—the larger the number of leaves—the more meaningful the results will be, though in any case interpreting them involves much calculating.

The ideal test, which provides an absolute count of all virus particles in a solution, was developed with bacteriophage. Like the test for TMV it is based on the fact that virus-infected cells will die. Phage-infected bacteria not only die but also disintegrate. If a solution containing a few hundred phage particles is applied to a thick, even lawn of bacteria growing in a dish of nutrient medium, a clear hole will shortly be formed in the turbid bacterial lawn wherever a phage particle has landed (Fig. 7). Each of these holes or "plaques," as they are called, is a circular area in which the bacteria have disintegrated. The plaques can easily be counted, and their number is equal to the phage particles in the sample of solution brought onto the dish, which is just what we wanted to know! With this trick, particles which are smaller than the ten-thousandth part of a millimeter are made "visible" to the naked eye. Don't forget, though, that it is not the particles themselves that we see, but only their effects.

Here is how the plaques are formed: A virus particle lands on the tightly packed bacterial lawn and infects one of the cells (the bacterial cells do not have to be damaged to be receptive as do the cells of the tobacco leaf). Within a few minutes the infected bacterium produces several hundred new phage particles, and then bursts, scattering phage all around the neighborhood. The new phage particles immediately infect further bacteria, in which many more phage are reproduced, and by now there will be several thousand descendants of the original particle. The process continues in ever widening circles

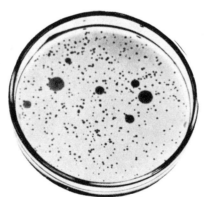

FIG. 7. Glass dish with bacterial lawn on solidified nutrient medium. Phage particles of different types have produced large (T_3) and small (T_2) holes in the bacterial growth.

until the stepwise production of billions of phage particles has destroyed so many bacteria that the place where
these used to be can be seen as a round hole.

To check on the accuracy of the plaque test, an equivalent sample of the test solution can be examined under
the electron microscope and the phage particles counted
directly, provided the solution was sufficiently concentrated and purified. Each type of phage has a characteristic shape (Fig. 14), and it is therefore quite feasible
to count them. The numbers obtained in this way check
very well with the results of the plaque test, thus proving
the reliability of the latter.

As intimated earlier, a variation of the plaque test has
now been worked out for animal-pathogenic viruses also.
Bacteria cannot be used, of course, since these viruses

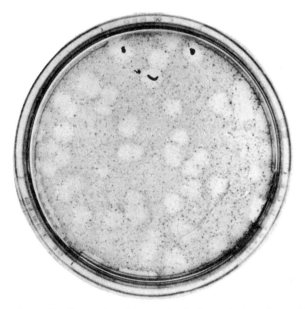

FIG. 8. Artificially produced layer of cells from chicken tissue. The
discolored spots are areas where the cells have been killed by
particles of the western equine encephalitis virus (WEE). (R. Dul-
becco, *Proc. Nat. Acad. Sci.*, 38 [1952], 747.)

require warm-blooded animal cells to grow in. The problem therefore was to induce animal cells to form a layer similar to the bacterial lawn. This proved difficult at first, but is now possible, and the viruses form discolored spots in the layer of tissue cells (Fig. 8). These spots, like those on the tobacco leaf, represent areas of dead cells. They are not completely disintegrated as are phage-infected bacterial cells. This test gives absolute indications of virus quantity if all the particles in the applied solution will find receptive cells, which is not necessarily the case. Still, the test is much more accurate than the leaf test for TMV.

Isolation

Just as it is necessary to work out a good quantitative test for each virus before attempting to isolate it, it is necessary to have the virus in isolated form before its structure and chemistry can be studied. Impurities in a virus preparation—usually disintegration products of the cells in which the virus was produced—make chemical experiments impossible, and it is just such chemical experiments which give the most interesting results. A pure virus preparation in the hands of the exact scientist is like a skeleton key which can be used to spy on the most subtle chemical secrets within the cell. Its use may be a little problematic, yet—perhaps for just this reason—it is certainly exciting.

A chemist might well consider the crystallizability of a substance to be sufficient proof of its purity, and, vice versa, everything that crystallizes he will be inclined to consider as a pure substance. Thus, when a crystalline form of TMV was produced more than twenty years ago, this automatically removed all doubts that the crystals, and therefore the virus, represented merely a chemical substance, not an organism. In those days no one would have dreamed of discussing an amorphous (noncrystallizable) virus preparation, be it the purest in the world, in terms describing it as a substance in the chemical sense. Thus it was actually an effect of no fundamental importance at all which focused the general attention on viruses and made them appear in a new light. That TMV would crystallize so obligingly may well be called one of the luckiest events in the biological sciences.

Since that time more has been learned about crystallization and purity, and ideas have changed. The crystalline form of a virus may not be pure, and a really pure preparation of active virus, on the other hand, may always successfully resist crystallization. It is now known that the ability of particles to aggregate into crystals depends on such chance factors as the regularity of their outer shape, the distribution of electrical charges on their surfaces, and so forth. Today it is merely a form of sport to tickle a virus preparation in various ingenious ways until, perhaps, it consents to fall into pretty crystals (Fig. 9). Since, however, the surface differences between infectious and noninfectious particles may be very minor,

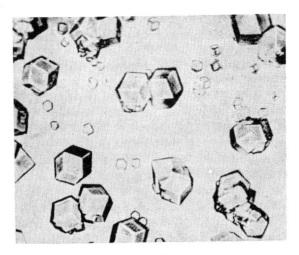

FIG. 9. Crystals of the "Bushy stunt" virus magnified about 300 times. These crystals, like the ones in Fig. 3, are made up of spherical virus particles, which, however, cannot be seen at the low magnification here. (F. C. Bawden, *Plant Viruses and Virus Diseases*, Waltham, Mass., 1950.)

the resulting crystals may well contain active particles side by side with some that were inactivated during the preparation. Without an absolute test there is no way of telling, and in this sense crystallization is not a reliable criterion of virus purity. This is, of all things, precisely the situation with TMV.

But if the ability to form crystals does not prove anything about substance vs. organism, what does? It is an interesting question and we have touched on it before. Viruses, like atoms and ordinary molecules, are static structures so long as they are on their own. A virus particle can only temporarily borrow a sham life from a real organism (a living cell). What the cell has and the virus particle must borrow, as we learned in Chapter II, is an autonomous system of chemical assembly lines. The chemical molecules which make up such a system are static in themselves but, in reacting with one another ceaselessly according to chemical laws, they work together to keep up and reproduce the whole system. In other words, in addition to a rather complex static organization in space, which a virus also has, a true organism like the cell possesses a dynamic organization in time; the term "organism" ought really to be reserved for structures like the latter.

Now we can return to the subject of virus purification. For any material to be separable from impurities, it must be physically or chemically different from these. Viruses usually fulfill this condition in two ways: differential solubility and rather high particle weight.

Solubility differences are utilized as follows: Viruses are usually not very soluble in water containing a lot of salt or a little acid. If some salt or acid is added to a virus solution which has been cleared of gross impurities by light centrifugation, then the virus cannot remain dissolved any longer and forms a sediment in the bottom of the test tube. Of course this sediment is not pure virus yet; it contains many other substances which also do not like salt or acid or which were simply pulled down along with the virus. All other materials, however—quite a large percentage of the impurities—remain dissolved in the fluid and can be poured off.

How can we be so sure that the virus really is in the sediment? Maybe there was not enough salt or acid added, or the virus couldn't take the treatment and has lost its infectivity. Here the biochemist has to use his artificial eye, the quantitative test, and, in fact, from now on this test must be applied after every step of the purification procedure to determine which of the fractions contains the active virus. There are often ten or twenty such fractions which must be tested, and it may well happen that the virus is inactivated during one of the steps, in which case the procedure has to start all over again with variations, until the proper procedure has been found.

Let us say the virus is in the sediment. Then this may be dissolved in water again, and the addition of various salts and acids repeated to get rid of more and more of the impurities. There is no limit to ingenious treatments and their skillful adaptation to the purpose in mind.

Finally, when alternate dissolving and precipitating do not help any more, and there still seem to be impurities, one may take advantage of the comparatively large particle weight of most viruses. (Sometimes, as in the case of bacteriophage, it may work out best to do this first.) A special high-speed centrifuge, called an ultracentrifuge, can rotate fast enough to draw solid sugar from a sugar-and-water solution. Virus particles, which are about 10,000 times bigger and heavier than sugar molecules, don't require such high speed, only 30,000–50,000 rotations per minute. Even at this rate a point on the rim of the turning mechanism is going round at approximately the speed of a bullet.

The virus solution is put into plastic tubes—glass would burst at this high speed—which are fitted into

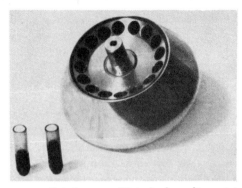

FIG. 10. Rotating part (Rotor) of an ultracentrifuge. Tubes containing virus solution fit into the holes.

the Rotor (Fig. 10), and the mad merry-go-round begins. After about an hour the machine is turned off; a solid deposit of pure virus—we hope—is found at the bottom of each tube. It may be pure virus, unless the solution contained other particles of the same or greater weight, in which case these will have been deposited along with the virus and must be separated from it by still other means.

What means? You might think that the end of the rope has been reached, but it hasn't. Particles of the same weight but different chemical structure may still have different electrical charges. In an electric field, between a positive and a negative pole, those particles with the highest charge will move most rapidly from one pole to the other. Imagine the situation: A direct current is passed through a solution containing particles of different charges, and immediately they begin their race. Soon they collect into groups according to their charge, and the longer the race continues, the more distinct the groups become. To give them plenty of time the race course is usually made of a narrow U-shaped tube.

It is even possible to "see" the different groups by making use of a well-known optical trick. I am sure everyone has, on occasion, observed air quivering above a hot roof or chimney. Air, of course, is invisible, but what you have seen was hot air entering cold air. What happens is that light rays are less deflected by hot air, which is not as dense as cold air. This causes the background distortion which we speak of as "quivering." The groups of particles in the U-shaped tube deflect light more strongly than the intervening water, and the resulting background distortions clearly indicate the position of each group. All that needs to be done now is to clamp off the tube between the groups, and there they sit, each in its own little trap, waiting to be tested to determine which is the virus.

The whole procedure above is called "electrophoresis" (literally "electric transport"). It is also used to test whether a preparation of charged particles is homogeneous or not. If the particles are of the same size, and they move at the same rate in the electric field, the chances are that they are of the same type. Electrophoresis has the advantage that it can be used with the most sensitive substances because it does not do them any harm. In this respect it is superior to the ultracentrifuge where the tight packing of the sediment may have critically harmful effects.

The ultracentrifuge, by the way, may also be used to check on the homogeneity of a virus preparation. Whereas electrophoresis separates particles into groups according to electric charge, centrifugation separates them according to weight. Particles which are equally heavy move away from the center of rotation at the same rate. Consequently a mixture of particles will be separated into groups according to weight during centrifugation. An optical apparatus attached to the ultracentrifuge (Fig. 11) makes it possible to "see" these groups in the same way as described in connection with electrophoresis. If centrifugation reveals only one group of particles they

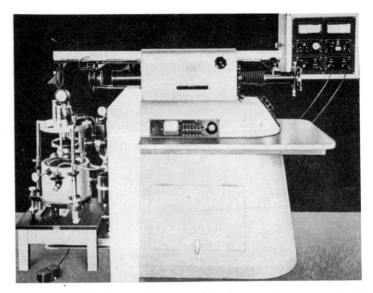

FIG. 11. An ultracentrifuge unit: left, the centrifuge proper, which is driven by compressed air, and is here shown open; right, the optical apparatus. (G. Schramm.)

must all belong to the same weight class, and the preparation is, in this respect, homogeneous.

From the rate of movement during electrophoresis it is possible to calculate the electrical charge per particle. Similarly, the weight per particle can be calculated from the rate of sedimentation. Such measurements and calculations also provide some clues about the particle's shape. For instance, it was known that TMV particles must be rod-shaped, not spherical, long before the invention of the electron microscope made it possible to look at them.

Once electrophoresis and ultracentrifugation have shown the virus preparation to be free of impurities, an attempt may be made to crystallize it. Usually this is done by again precipitating it with salt, but very slowly and carefully this time, and at near the freezing point. If the virus precipitates too suddenly, it is usually amorphous. If given plenty of time—possibly several days—the virus may oblige and form pretty crystals at the bottom of the flask.

Chemical description

Once the virus has been purified, the biochemist is apt to take the precious stuff, shove it in a glass tube, and burn it up. No, he hasn't lost his wits in the long struggle for pure virus; he is simply making use of the fact that oxidation changes all organic substances, including viruses, into simple compounds such as carbon dioxide, water, ammonia, phosphoric acid, sulphuric acid, and so forth. The sample was carefully weighed before oxidation, and the substances derived from it are weighed again. Now it is easy to calculate the percentages of the various elements—carbon, hydrogen, nitrogen, phosphorus, sulfur, and so forth—in the original material. Other chemical tests provide clues about the way in which the atoms of these elements are put together forming certain structural subunits of the material under investigation, whereby it can be roughly classified. Finally, the biochemist may try to figure out how these structural subunits are arranged in the total structure.

All this takes a long time, but we can rush to the conclusion which has been reached through innumerable experiments performed with many virus types: Viruses always consist of two main components, "protein" and "nucleic acid" (so called because it was first found in cell nuclei). There is no virus without protein and nucleic acid, and many virus types consist of nothing but these two substances.

Protein and nucleic acid however exist in many forms. In fact the principle of their construction makes almost infinite variations possible. A molecule of each is made up of an enormous number of chemically characteristic building blocks; each of these building blocks can mesh with others of its own kind in certain ways to form the superstructures which we then call protein or nucleic acid. How the cell goes about combining simple building blocks into complex structures was discussed in Chapter II.

The building blocks which go to make up protein are called "amino acids." They usually consist of a relatively small number of carbon, hydrogen, nitrogen, oxygen, and, possibly, sulphur atoms. In the structure of each amino acid there are at least two places at which a chemical bond may be formed linking it to another one. The simplest superstructures they can form are therefore chains. To get an idea of the number of combinations such a system makes possible, let us assume for a moment that there are only four different amino acids available, *A, B, C,* and *D,* and see how many four-link chains we can make of them. First of all we use only one of the four types, *AAAA, BBBB,* and so forth. Then we can add one of the others, which leads to *BAAA, ABBB, ABAA,* and so forth. When all of these possibilities are exhausted, we can add the third, and finally the fourth type, and wind up with *ABCD, ACBD, DCBA,* and so forth. You can see what an astonishing variety of combinations is possible using only four different links. For proteins, however, more than twenty different amino acids are available, and protein chains contain not four links but hundreds or thousands. The possible combinations here reach astronomical numbers. We cannot even imagine such numbers, and only a mathematician can calculate them. Some amino acids even have three or more places at which they can intermesh so that the final structure of a protein is not just simple chains but a complex three-dimensional network. Now even the mathematician will have to give up.

Theoretically, then, an inconceivably great number of protein molecules can be constructed. However, a particular protein molecule has its particular characteristics, and the chemist has various means of distinguishing one from another. Particle charge and particle weight can be determined by electrophoresis and centrifugation. The protein can be injected into a suitable warm-blooded animal, where it will induce the formation of antibodies which will combine exclusively with the type of protein that induced them. This reaction in its various forms— one of them is the Wassermann reaction—is so specific that it can be widely used for the characterization of proteins. Furthermore it is possible to split up a given protein into its component amino acids, so that at least the gross composition can be ascertained. The final problem is of course to determine the order of the components in any particular protein. This enormous task, called fine-structure analysis, is being worked on by many researchers in various laboratories.

So much for proteins. The other major component of viruses, nucleic acid, seems in some ways to be a simpler structure. It is composed of just four different building blocks, called nucleotides, which combine in chains only. Remember, however, how many combinations are possible with only the four letters A, B, C, and D, especially where each of them may occur more than a thousand times in the chain. Each of these nucleotides consists of three distinct components: one molecule "base," one molecule "sugar," and one molecule "phosphoric acid." They are combined like this:

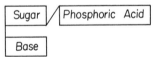

Some nucleotides contain a sugar called "ribose" and others contain "desoxyribose." However, a given nucleic acid chain will have only the one or the other type of sugar, so that there are two main classes of nucleic acid: ribonucleic acid (RNA) and desoxyribonucleic acid (DNA). Cells contain both RNA and DNA, but virus particles seem always to have only one or the other. RNA occurs in most plant and animal viruses, whereas bacteriophage have DNA.

The nucleotides in a given nucleic acid chain are all alike not only with respect to their sugar component. The same is also true for the phosphoric acid. There are, however, different bases. DNA, for instance, contains four kinds. Let us draw another picture: We will designate the bases with the first letters of their names—*A* for adenine, *C* for cytosine, *G* for guanine, and *T* for thymine. The sugar will be a vertical line, and the phosphoric acid an angle. Then we have the following four different kinds of nucleotides to build DNS chains from:

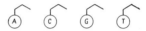

Adding to the picture the fact that the phosphoric acid can form a link between nucleotides by reaching from its own sugar molecule to a neighboring one, we simply have to shove together symbols like those above in order to obtain a real drawing of a DNS chain:

.... Ⓒ Ⓣ Ⓐ Ⓐ Ⓖ Ⓐ Ⓣ Ⓣ ....

Speculation

Before we get involved in further details, let us stop at this point to consider the significance of the facts we already know. Why is information about viruses so especially exciting? Viruses are made of protein and nucleic acid. Where else do we find something comparable? The answer is: in the nuclei of cells, where there are long, threadlike structures called chromosomes. These chromosomes also consist of protein and nucleic acid, and at each division of the cell an exact copy of each chromosome is produced. We know that they are exact copies because, in relation to viruses, chromosomes are enormous and their special structural characteristics can actually be seen under the microscope. On the basis of innumerable different experiments it has long been assumed that the microscopically visible chromosomes consist of many smaller distinct units, called genes (which are not visible). Genes are the hereditary factors of the organism; they are responsible for transferring its characteristics from one generation to the next.

Are genes, like viruses, self-reproducing? It would be very nice to think so, for the following reason: If you will remember in Chapter II we discussed the chemical assembly lines which operate in the cell. The workers on these assembly lines are enzymes, and their job is to act as middlemen in the stepwise synthesis of various substances the cell needs. Among the substances which the cell needs are, of course, the enzymes themselves. Consequently we have to imagine the cell containing special enzymes to make its enzymes, and more enzymes to make the special enzymes, and so forth. Where does it all end, and how do we get a closed and self-sufficient cycle? Somewhere we have to imagine a "short-circuit," and for this job the gene has been elected.

It is not at all arbitrary to think of the gene as the link which closes the chain. We know that genes act as hereditary factors by determining the chemical possibilities of the cell and its descendants. This is where enzymes come in again: It is known that each gene somehow sees to it that a particular enzyme is formed. Should the structure of a particular gene in the cell be changed (mutation) or destroyed, then the corresponding enzyme, for the correct synthesis of which the gene was responsible, is not produced any more. As a result, a certain chemical process in the cell no longer takes place. In other words, all the genes a cell may treasure represent an invaluable archive in which every detail of the cell's means for chemical performances is deposited in "written" form. Obviously, then, it is most important that each gene be copied exactly at each cell division. If we now assume that all those genes can make copies of themselves (without each requiring its own special "copying enzyme"), then the cycle would be closed at the only really logical place.

Nobody has ever seen genes, unfortunately, much less obtained them in pure form. We can, however, study viruses; they are chemically closely related to genes and do possess the ability to instigate in cells the making of exact copies of themselves. They have even, occasionally, been spoken of as "vagrant genes," though this turned out to be misleading because, as we shall see, some viruses possess several genes. In any case viruses seem to have enough in common with genes so that information about virus reproduction is likely to give us important clues about the very trick by which the synthetic activities of chemical systems can be made to work around in a circle—that is, the trick which causes them to *live!* Since the virus actually enters the chemical cycle of the cell and reproduces in it, we have the means now of opening up that cycle just at the point which normally insures that it is closed, without blocking at the same time the all-important copying mechanism which operates at this same point.

Since viruses, and presumably also genes, consist of protein and nucleic acid, one tried at first, very optimistically, to guess at the copying mechanism from the general structure of these two components, about which too little was known. Models were visualized which were to show that protein and nucleic acid under proper conditions just can't help making copies of themselves (or possibly of each other). The structure to be copied merely had to catch free building-blocks—amino acids or nucleotides, which the cell always provides—and to line these up in a way mirroring the arrangement of its own building blocks. All that was then necessary was for some sewing machine to tie securely together the aligned elements. Very nice, but unfortunately all the early models which were constructed to illustrate such a system somehow resembled the *perpetuum mobile:* They wouldn't work. Nevertheless, some variation of this kind of reproductive system is still favored. It is called a template mechanism because the structure to be reproduced is, itself, the unchanging die stamp or mold from which copies are made. The system is "autocatalytic" if each new copy is a new template as well, helping with the disking out of further copies. Everything is done by the multiplying structure itself. There is no outside catalyst required to make the copy. An autocatalytic reproductive system obviously results in a geometric increase in the number of new structures. A more complicated autocatalytic system would involve continuous alternation between a "negative" and a "positive" of the structure which is in the process of being copied. Another possibility is that the original structure makes one negative from which all further copies are then produced as prints. This would no longer be an autocatalytic process, though; the number of copies could only increase arithmetically.

Before we leave these preliminary speculations, there is one more point to show that they are not at all idle speculations: Hundreds of enzymes are known which can change all kinds of materials into other materials, but we don't know a single enzyme which can make real protein out of amino acids, or nucleic acid of specific structure from nucleotides. Yet no other materials are synthesized so frequently in nature. Every spring, when the leaves come out on the trees, millions and millions of tons of protein and nucleic acid are produced in a very short time—and we don't know how. There can be no doubt that protein biosynthesis and nucleic acid biosynthesis carry each other's secrets.

Looking at pictures

In the laboratory, looking at virus particles comes last, after the preparation has been purified and chemically characterized. It seemed fitting, therefore, to save the pictures of viruses for the end of the chapter, as a sort of reward for the reader who has fought his way through this far.

Here is the polio virus in crystalline and free form (Figs. 12 and 13) and bacteriophage (Fig. 14). We immediately notice the peculiar phage "tail," which may be short and rigid as in phage $T2$ (Fig. 14) or long and flexible as in $T5$ (Fig. 19). Sometimes the tail is rudimentary, but no phage type seems to lack it entirely. For a long time the function of this member was unknown. The term "tail" implied that it was attached to the "back" end of the particle, and maybe some investigators

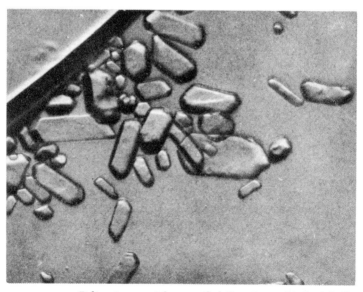

FIG. 12. Polio virus crystals magnified 800 times. (F. L. Schaffer and C. E. Schwerdt, *Proc. Nat. Acad. Sci.*, 41 [1955], 1020.)

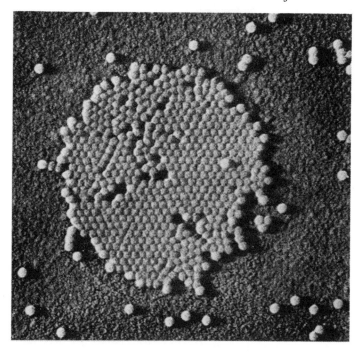

FIG. 13. Spherical particles of polio virus seen under the electron microscope (magnified 83,000 times). The particles here happened to aggregate in such a way that they could form the first layer in a crystal. Many such layers, one on top of the other, make up crystals, as in Fig. 12. (C. E. Schwerdt *et al.*, *Proc. Soc. Exper. Biol. and Med.*, 86 [1954], 310.)

privately considered whether it might not serve for locomotion. As we know, however, viruses have no chemical assembly lines of their own from which they could derive the energy to move. Considering the way a phage particle attacks its host cell, the "tail" is in "front," if anywhere, though the terms front and back do not have much meaning with virus particles. Spheric virus particles like polio (Fig. 13) or tobacco necrosis (Fig. 3) make this fairly obvious. But even if there are two ends to a particle like the rod of TMV (Fig. 15) or the thread

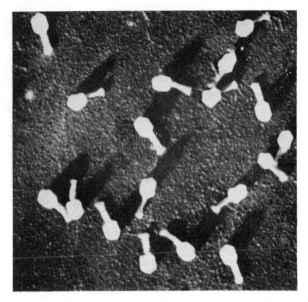

FIG. 14. Bacteriophage *T2* seen under the electron microscope (magnified 37,000 times). Each of these particles can produce a plaque in a bacterial lawn, and so become directly "visible." (R. M. Herriott and J. L. Barlow, *J. Gen. Physiol.*, 36 [1953], 17.)

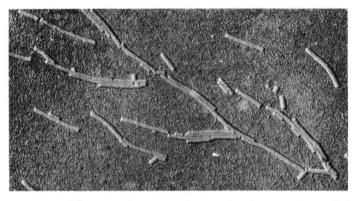

FIG. 15. Electron microscope photograph of TMV (magnified about 50,000 times). The particles are about to aggregate into bundles. When the bundles are thick enough, they appear as the crystalline needles of Fig. 2. (G. Schramm.)

of potato Y (Fig. 16), neither one deserves any preference.

So much for looking at virus particles. In the next chapter we are going to study the particle in action, and we will see how temporary is its outer form. What we refer to as "the virus particle" is actually only a snapshot from a drama with continually changing scenes. The snapshot naturally cannot tell us much about the plot.

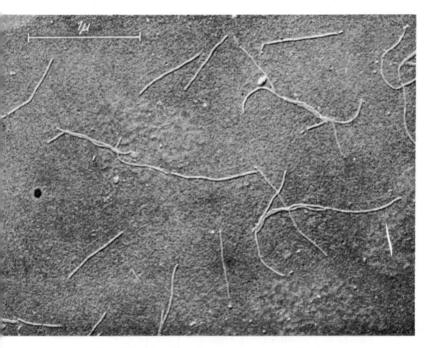

FIG. 16. Threadlike particles of potato Y Virus, with a line representing $\frac{1}{1000}$ millimeter drawn in for comparison (magnified 30,000 times). (G. Schramm.)

IV. *The Virus and the Cell*

Basic difference between virus and a living organism

Facing any fairly complicated state of affairs in science, not even the most inspired genius will be able to dream up an experiment which once and for all decides the issue. The mechanism of virus reproduction is probably more than a little complicated; many inspired men had to do series upon series of experiments without achieving more each time than throwing narrow beams of light from slightly different angles on the problems. If darkness is to become lucid, we must follow their experiments. The reader may draw consolation from the fact that he, at least, is not pressed for thinking up experiments to answer specific questions, for figuring out the meaning of their usually unexpected results, and for planning more experiments to straighten out apparent paradoxes.

In the following, we shall discuss mostly experiments done with phage. The reason is that phage particles, as will be remembered, can be counted most easily and accurately, which makes results most clear-cut. The first experiments will remind us once more of the conditions necessary for virus reproduction as compared with those required for the multiplication of a living organism like the bacterial cell.

If bacterial cells are kept in a weak salt solution, they do not, of course, multiply, because the old cells cannot make new ones just from salt. On the other hand, no harm occurs to the original cells either; they stay alive for a long time. This can easily be proven by taking measured samples of the cell suspension at regular intervals and spreading them on solidified nutrient medium in a Petri dish. (The solidifying medium is called "agar" and such dishes are referred to as "agar plates.") Soon after landing on the agar, each living cell begins to take up nutrients and to produce daughter cells. The daughter cells all stay close together, and presently there will be enough of them so that they can be seen with the naked eye (Fig. 17). Such a group of cells, all derived from a single cell, is called a colony. The more living cells there were in the test sample, the more colonies there will be on the agar plate. So long as equal samples of the bacterial suspension in saline continue to produce the same number of colonies, we can be sure that none of the suspended cells has died of hunger or suffered any other misfortune.

A similar experiment with phage particles in a salt

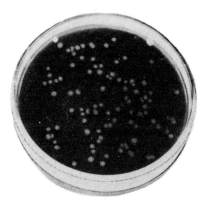

FIG. 17. Individual bacterial colonies on an agar plate.

solution leads to the same result. Obviously the phage particles cannot multiply in the salt solution; on the other hand, they are not "inactivated"—they do not lose the *ability* to multiply. Equal samples of this phage suspension continue for weeks and months to produce the same number of plaques in a bacterial lawn. As we know, each plaque derives from a single phage particle which has produced millions of descendants; it is a phage colony, in other words, quite analogous to the bacterial colony.

Now let us take another bacterial salt-water suspension and add some suitable nutrients, for example, meat extract. We again take samples of the suspension at regular intervals to make colony counts, and now we find that the number of colonies increases rapidly. Why? Because the cells are multiplying in the solution which now contains nutrients. The average time it takes one cell to make one division can be calculated from the rate of increase in the number of colonies. If a sample taken at time t_2 produces twice as many colonies as a sample taken at time t_1, then the time difference $t_2 - t_1$ equals the average time per cell division. With a fresh culture it always takes the same length of time for a given number of colonies to double. Such cultures are said to increase "geometrically."

If meat extract is added to the phage suspension, nothing changes at all. Samples taken at intervals always produce the same number of plaques. The phage particles do not multiply even though nutrients are supplied.

Here we seem to have discovered a very remarkable difference between virus and cell. But wait, is it really significant? We have not excluded the possibility that bacteria eat nutrients but that viruses have to eat bacteria. We had better do another experiment. This time we will add bacteria to the phage suspension in salt water. This ought to supply the virus with all it needs to grow and multiply.

No sooner said than done, but nothing happens; the plaque test shows no increase in phage particles. Now there is only one more possibility. We offer bacteria to the phage and nutrients to the bacteria. These are the conditions which actually exist on the agar plate used for plaque tests. There we have a (solidified) nutrient medium which keeps the bacteria going, on which in turn the phage happily multiplies. Could we guess, though, that the phage particles would not be happy with bacteria alone?

Anyway, we perform the experiment: a suspension of phage in salt water, add bacteria, add meat extract, and behold—samples taken at intervals produce more and more plaques on the test plate. Under these conditions the number of phage particles increases; they multiply in the suspension.

Now, what have we proven? It is not enough to offer living bacteria to the phage; the bacteria must also be stimulated, by the addition of nutrients, to set their chemical assembly lines in motion as if they themselves were going to increase. "As if" is the significant phrase here. Actually the chemical assembly lines run at full speed (as proven by all kinds of biochemical experiments, which we won't discuss here), but not a single bacterial division takes place nor ever will. Samples of the phage-bacteria-nutrient mixture no longer produce a single bacterial colony, although without the phage there should be thousands. Why then all this fuss with the chemical machinery of the cells working so hard? Obviously to make more phage! Phage don't know what to do with more substances or materials. For their multiplication they require running assembly lines which they find in working cells only. Forced by the infecting phage particle, the bacterial cell, strangely enough, gives up the production of material for new bacterial cells and makes new phage particles instead.

The situation, far from being straightforward, is clearly

going to lead us into all kinds of intricacies. It is similar with all other viruses, but it is not always so easy to design experiments to prove it.

Rest, activity, rest: the reproductive cycle

The next questions we would like to have answered are: How does phage reproduction take place *in time*, and how many particles are produced per infected bacterial cell? Both questions can be answered with one clever experiment.

We take a suspension of bacteria in nutrient broth and determine by the colony count exactly how many cells it contains. (This could also be done under the microscope with a counting chamber, the way blood counts are done in a hospital.) Then we infect every bacterial cell in the suspension simply by adding enough phage particles. Now we have a suspension of infected cells of known number. We immediately start taking samples, one every minute, for the usual plaque test.

Result: On the first agar plates the number of plaques corresponds exactly to the number of infected cells in the suspension. This is to be expected because every infected cell, just like a free phage particle, must produce a single plaque in the bacterial lawn. It does not matter whether the first bacterium is infected in the lawn on the test plate (as is the case where *free* particles are being counted) or whether the infection takes place earlier, as in the experiment here. The test plates made during the first minutes show that the number of bacteria in the suspension does not change. Counting under the microscope would give the same result, but a bacterial colony count would not be possible, because, as we know, phage-infected cells no longer form colonies.

But then suddenly a change in the number of plaques takes place; the twentieth plate (made exactly twenty minutes after infection) definitely shows more plaques than all the previous ones. On the following plates the number of plaques increases rapidly until a new level is reached about five plates (five minutes) later. From now on the number of plaques remains constant again, but it surpasses that on the first plates by several hundred.

What happens in the suspension of phage-infected cells between the twentieth and the twenty-fifth minute? Watching it through the microscope we observe that from the twentieth minute on, the number of bacteria rapidly decreases. One can actually see the cells burst and disintegrate. From the parallel increase of the plaque count on the plates we have to conclude that upon bursting the cells must be scattering newly made phage particles in the suspending fluid, whereas up to that moment these particles must have been stored within the cells. A sample of the fluid taken at this time contains not only infected cells but also free virus particles, each of which can now start a plaque of its own on the test plate.

The rapid increase in the number of plaques shows that the cells all burst within a very short time span (five minutes). When the last cell has scattered its contents, the number of plaques no longer increases; from then on the suspension contains only free phage particles. These, now that they are on their own, can no longer multiply, and their number therefore remains constant.

We may find that for each plaque counted before the twentieth minute there will now be, on the average, 250 additional plaques. This means that each infected cell has produced an average of 250 new phage particles. It makes no difference, incidentally, whether the cell was infected by only one phage particle, or several at the same time.

The disintegration of the bacterium and the simultaneous scattering of new virus particles is called "lysis." The time it takes a bacterium to produce the average number of 250 new phage particles—the period between infection and lysis, in other words—is called the "latent period." This latent period is characteristic for each phage type. Some phage types have a long latent period, for example, forty-five minutes, while for others it may be as short as thirteen minutes. Within this latent period the entire reproductive cycle of the phage particle takes place.

Before its meeting with a suitable bacterial cell, the phage particle was an inert substance, and it might have remained that way forever. Given the opportunity of entering a living cell, however, the phage particle multiplies a hundredfold within a few minutes. Each of the descendants is exactly like the original particle, also with respect to the quality of inertness, until, by chance, it meets a fresh host cell, in which case it can start the reproductive cycle again. Thus all virus particles vacillate between a period of rest, which may be of any length, and a short phase of activity.

No wonder the first researchers thought it wouldn't take them long to find out all about virus reproduction! After all, how much can happen in the few minutes it takes a phage particle to multiply a hundredfold? Years of research have now shown that quite a lot can happen, and the whole process is, by no means, entirely understood yet.

Experimental subdivision of the reproductive cycle

Now we know that the interesting steps of virus reproduction all take place between infection of the bacterial cell and its lysis; we can therefore try to subdivide this latent period further in order to study it better. After we have taken it apart, and carefully looked at the various phases, we can attempt to put it together again into a more meaningful whole.

Experimental subdivision of the reproductive cycle: first meeting between virus and host cell

Perhaps some readers have been wondering how virus and cell ever get together since in most cases neither of them can move. In describing the preceding experiment we slyly evaded this problem by saying that bacteria are infected "simply" by adding phage.

Injury.—With plant viruses there is no special problem. In the discussion of test methods for viruses it was mentioned that an injury makes plant cells receptive to the virus. In nature there is plenty of opportunity for such injuries to occur. The wind, moving a mosaic-diseased plant so that its leaves rub against a healthy plant, may be sufficient to infect the latter. The chewing and boring of insects often serves to spread viruses from plant to plant. Once a virus particle has found a way through the plant cell wall, its descendants will have no trouble infecting the whole organism. Only toward the outside are plant cells protected by the tough cell wall; inside, the cells are all connected by fine pores in the separating walls, and the viruses can be carried everywhere by the plant sap.

Collision.—The story is quite different for viruses which attack single cells such as bacteria. There won't be any insects to bore holes into them. Generally such organisms are too small to be subject to mechanical injury in their natural habitat. A few experiments will show how phage and bacteria do, nevertheless, make a durable contact.

We take a bacterial suspension in saline which looks turbid because of the many cells it contains, and centrifuge it at about 3,000 r.p.m. (revolutions per minute), a relatively low speed of rotation. After five minutes we stop the centrifuge. It is obvious even to the naked eye that the liquid is quite clear, and there is a sediment of tightly packed bacteria at the bottom of the tube. The bacterial cells are heavy enough so that they are pulled down even by this moderate centrifugal force.

If we now repeat the experiment with phage (or other viruses) the bottom of the tube stays quite free of sediment, and a test shows that the virus particles remain equally distributed throughout the liquid. Virus particles are too light for the weak centrifugal force to pull them down.

Now let us mix the bacterial and phage suspensions, wait a few minutes, and then centrifuge again at 3,000 r.p.m. The bacterial cells sink, as expected, but now the phage particles go along. The plaque test reveals that only a very small percentage of phage has remained suspended in the liquid. This shows that the phage particles must actually stick to the bacteria, once they happen to collide. The collisions as such are accidental. They are caused by the Brownian (thermal) motion of the water molecules in the suspension which push around the virus particles as well as the bacteria.

Adsorption.—This "sticking" of the virus to the host cell is called "adsorption." It can easily be proven that adsorption precedes, and is a prerequisite for, infection. If the sediment of bacteria with adhering phage particles is mixed up again in nutrient solution, then the bacterial cells will burst after the usual latent period and scatter great numbers of newly produced phage. In other words, the bacteria were actually infected.

If the same experiment is repeated with another phage type but the same bacterial type, or vice versa, it may easily happen that the phage particles will not stick to the bacteria; the bacteria alone sink during centrifugation and the phage remain suspended in the fluid. In such cases the bacteria are not infected and they can continue to live and happily multiply. This proves again that adsorption must precede infection. It also proves that there is no "general stickiness" of bacteria which permits phage to adhere; rather we are dealing with specific attractions between certain cell types and certain virus types. As it turns out, every virus type has a limited "host range" of cell types by which it is adsorbed and reproduced; similarly each cell type can only be infected by certain virus types and not by others.

Can only live bacteria, with functioning assembly lines, adsorb phage? The question can easily be answered by the following experiment: Bacterial cells are killed by heat or chemicals and suspended in a salt-water solution. Phage of a type known to adsorb these cells when they are alive are added. Centrifugation proves that, even though they are dead, these bacteria still adsorb phage. The centrifuged liquid hardly contains any more phage particles; they must have been pulled down into the sediment along with the dead cells. If this sediment, consisting of dead cells and adhering virus particles, is mixed up again in nutrient solution, nothing happens. The cells will never burst and liberate new phage particles; "killing" the bacteria means destroying their chemical assembly lines, without which no new virus can be produced.

The dead cells do not make any new virus, but usually they do not let go of the particles which adhere to them. No matter what means are tried, the phage particles cannot be retrieved in active form; they are stuck for good and can never infect another cell. Samples of dead bacteria and phage produce hardly any plaques on a test plate. The few plaques which are found are due to phage particles which, at the time the sample was taken, had not yet been adsorbed by a dead cell.

It is possible to prove, with other similar experiments, that a live or dead bacterial cell can adsorb not just one phage particle but many, possibly hundreds. This is most important because it provides the opportunity to infect one cell with several different viruses and study the effects.

Receptor substances.—Since viruses can attach even

to dead cells, there must be some sort of "receptor" sub-stance in the cell wall which determines whether a certain virus is adsorbed or not. By various chemical means such substances can actually be extracted from the cell, and the extract will inactivate those types of phage which are infectious for the original cells, because the receptors, even in solution, still combine irreversibly with the virus particles as they did when they formed part of the intact cell wall. This effect provides the test necessary for any attempt to purify receptor substances. In order to prove its specificity, one makes similar extracts from cell types which do not adsorb the virus type in question. Such extracts, for lack of receptor-active material, in theory should not inactivate the virus—and they won't in fact.

The procedure for purifying an extracted receptor substance is similar to the method for obtaining a pure virus preparation. After every step in the purification procedure a sample is quantitatively tested against a known amount of virus. The larger the percentage of virus which is inactivated under fixed conditions, the more receptor substance must have been in the test sample. A material is finally obtained which, even when it is very dilute, inactivates a large amount of virus. Ultracentrifuge and electrophoresis show that the material is homogeneous; it must be pure receptor substance, having a specific affinity for the phage type used in the tests.

All the receptor substances isolated so far have certain characteristics in common: their particle weight is fairly high, about similar to that of viruses; they consist of proteins, fats, and various sugars combined into giant molecules; unlike viruses, the receptor substances do not contain nucleic acid. Figure 18 shows the particles of a receptor substance isolated from coli bacteria, a type of bacterium normally found in the human large intestine. As you can see, the particles of this receptor substance are spherical; their diameter is 0.00003 millimeters. Both

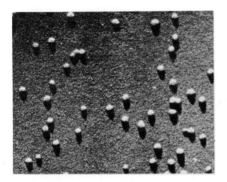

FIG. 18. Spherical particles of the receptor substance for phage T_5 (magnified
60,000 times). (W. Weidel and E. Kellenberger, *Biochim. et biophys. Acta*, 17
[1955], 1.)

of these facts were known from ultracentrifuge measurements even before the substance was isolated and photo-
graphed under the electron microscope.

The affinity of this receptor substance is directed
towards the phage T_5 particles of Figure 19, which, of
course, are infectious for coli bacteria. What happens
when some of the T_5 receptor substance is added to a
suspension of T_5 can be seen in Figure 20. We find one
particle of receptor substance attached to the tip of each
phage "tail." From the test we know that these phage
particles are now unable to multiply. The reason must be
that they cannot rid themselves from the receptor molecule blocking their "tail" tip, and consequently are unable to attach to a host cell. Normally, therefore, the
phage must attach to the cell with the tip of its "tail," and,
of course, at a spot where a receptor molecule is built
into the cell wall. In Figure 21 we can see that this is
true. Two bacterial cells are shown to which many
phage particles were adsorbed at the same time. The
phages do adhere with their "tail" tips, whereas the
"heads" stand away from the cell.

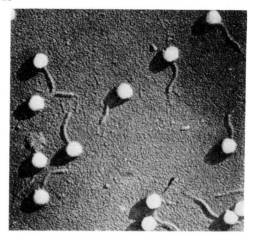

FIG. 19. Particles of bacteriophage *T5* (magnified 60,000 times). (W. Weidel and E. Kellenberger.)

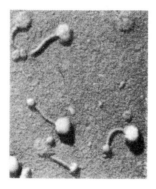

FIG. 20. *T5* particles inactivated by specific bacterial receptor substance (Fig. 18). Magnified 60,000 times. A particle of receptor substance adheres to each "tail" tip, thus blocking the attaching organ of the phage. (W. Weidel and E. Kellenberger.)

The reaction between receptor particle and "tail" tip must involve the formation of chemical bonds which firmly join the two components once they have come in contact. Since the reaction is also highly specific, the surfaces of the two structures must fit together like left and right hand when they are folded. Each type of phage has to have its own specially constructed receptor substance built into the wall of the cell which is to be infected. Where several different types of phage are infectious for the same cell, the wall of that cell is actually a mosaic of receptor substances, which are

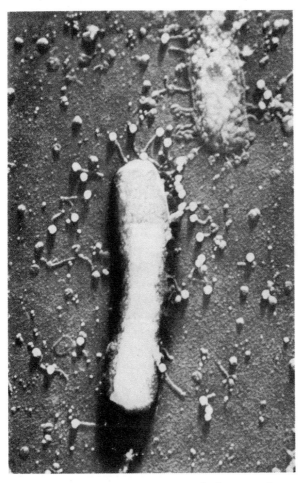

FIG. 21. Two cells of *Mycobacterium* with phage particles attached. Note that the particles adhere to the cell wall with the tips of their "tails." (G. Penso, "Virus and Cell," Sixth Internatl. Cong. for Microbiology, Rome, 1953.)

chemically different, and each is specific for one phage type. Those studying phage are now trying to find out how the specificity of this reaction is related to the chemical structures of "tail" tip and receptor molecule. Since both are highly complex structures, this is a large order.

Virus-resistant cells and their origin.—Why the cell is foolish enough to synthesize receptor substances at all is still a mystery. Without them it is both safe from virus attack and perfectly functional, as the following experiment proves.

A test plate is infected with not just a few hundred phage particles but so many that the bacterial lawn is completely destroyed. No individual plaques can be seen because they all overlap; only the bare nutrient agar remains as one giant plaque. If the plate is then kept for a while still in the incubator, a curious thing happens: individual bacterial colonies appear on the nutrient agar and grow rapidly. Here they are, in the midst of billions of phage particles, and it doesn't bother them a bit. Close examination of these bacteria proves that they are not contaminants from the air; they are descendants of the original cells, most of which were recently massacred on the plate by the phages. These bacteria are, however, completely phage-resistant. The centrifuge experiment reveals the reason: they no longer adsorb the phage type which destroyed their forebears, nor do they yield an extract which inactivates the phage. In other words, they no longer make that specific receptor substance, and neither will any of their descendants. From a biochemical point of view we might say that the assembly lines in these cells have been changed so that the particular receptor substance is not on these cells' list of synthetic products any more. Perhaps something else, harmless, is made instead; in any case the cells seem to get on perfectly well. Why, then, do not all bacteria give up the suicidal manufacture of receptor substances?

When we phrase the question in this way, we imply some sort of purposeful reaction to its environment on the part of the cell: it meets a dangerous enemy and responds with a defense mechanism. But this assumption is entirely wrong. Actually the change from susceptibility to resistance happens quite accidentally and spontaneously. There needs to be no meeting with the enemy; the change may occur in cells which never came in contact with phage. It happens rarely, however; among very large numbers of phage-susceptible cells there will never be more than a few which have suddenly given up the production of a certain receptor substance. In our experiment, these few remain on the test plate, and, when all their relatives have succumbed to the phages, they grow into the colonies which can soon be seen.

A spontaneous change in the chemical assembly lines which is permanent—that is to say, which is passed on from generation to generation—is called a mutation. The bacteria which have become virus-resistant are "mutants" because they arose, by mutation, from virus-susceptible cells.

The reader may find it difficult to believe that such a seemingly reasonable adjustment of the cell from virus-susceptibility to virus-resistance should be due to blind chance. It seems much easier to imagine the environment inducing changes in the organism than it is to think of the organism changing to suit environments which may not —or not yet—exist. Nevertheless the latter is the case. We can be absolutely sure that, for example, at the time of the pharaohs and even earlier, when chemical therapy had certainly not yet been invented, there were already bacteria arising spontaneously which would have been immune to the antibiotics of our time. Such bacteria are not new today, and they are not due to our use of antibiotics in the treatment of bacterial diseases. However, antibiotic-resistant bacteria had no particular advantage in a world which knew nothing of antibiotics. Nowadays, on the contrary, such resistant bacteria have considerable "selective advantage." Thus twenty years ago, in the early days of chemical therapy, gonorrhea used to be cured with sulfanilamide. This treatment does not work any more, not because the Gonococci have gotten used to the poison, but because, since its use, only those Gonococci which happened to evolve a system of assembly lines that cannot be blocked by the poison have had a chance to survive. Originally there were few of these, but they alone were chosen for survival. They have been "selected," and the means of their selection (though not the cause of their existence) was the sulfanilamide, which has consequently lost its usefulness in the treatment of gonorrhea.

No matter how reasonable and purposeful they may seem, the forces we have watched in action here are blind mutation and mechanical selection. Anyone who refuses to believe this—as the Russian geneticist Lysenko long did—is sacrificing evidence to prejudice.

By now it should be obvious that phages would not be very useful weapons in the fight against bacterial disease, as some readers may have hoped. Let us assume a typhus patient is treated with typhus phages. To be sure, the susceptible bacteria will be largely destroyed (though it might be difficult to catch each and every one of them with a phage). In any case, the few phage-resistant mutants, which undoubtedly exist, will remain; these will immediately increase in numbers, and since they are just as vicious as the phage-susceptible cells, the typhus patient will still be sick. When phages were first discovered about fifty years ago, phage therapy was actually tried. Today we understand why it failed.

A review of the preceding section will show that the seemingly simple problem of phage adsorption has led us to some rather far-reaching conclusions. This is as it should be, for there are no isolated facts. If it ever seems so, it is likely that somewhere or other the most important point has been overlooked.

The adsorption of many animal viruses is similar to that of phages. Here, too, receptor molecules must be built into the host's cell wall to attach the virus. The chemistry of some of these receptors has been intensively studied, but in this case as well the relationship of structure and function is still an open question.

Virus particles escape a trap.—We mentioned the ability of certain viruses to clump red blood cells when we were discussing quantitative tests. This phenomenon is of interest here since adsorption is involved. The red blood cells contain receptors for the viruses in question. Since, unlike phage particles, these viruses are spherical, they can attach at any point of their surface to the receptor substance. A single virus particle can form a bridge between two red blood cells by attaching to both of them, and since each blood cell can adsorb many of the relatively tiny particles, bridges are formed in all directions. Soon so many red blood cells have been glued together that the resulting clump can be seen with the naked eye.

Now, a red blood cell is not a complete and self-sufficient cell; it lacks almost all chemical assembly lines and is fated to die soon. Consequently it cannot make any new virus. A virus particle adsorbed to a red blood cell would therefore seem to be just as hopelessly trapped as the phage particle which has gotten stuck to a dead bacterium. In fact you would expect animal viruses coursing through the body—which is full of blood and even free receptor substance dissolved in the plasma—to run into this trap all the time. Unfortunately there is an escape, or we would scarcely have to worry about virus diseases.

If clumped red blood cells are allowed to stand for a while they will separate, and these same cells will never again form clumps. Fresh blood cells added to the mixture are still agglutinated, but will also separate after an interval. Each time a clump spontaneously separates, the virus, which had been adsorbed, is freed without having been changed in any way. What happens is that the virus itself destroys the receptor substance to which it was attached; it digests the receptor, and, in each case, leaves red blood cells which are free of receptor substances and can therefore no longer be agglutinated by viruses.

The viruses we are discussing are so constructed, in other words, that they can escape any trap set for them by their blind affinity for receptor substances. If we now consider that the cytoplasm of the host cell, where new viruses are made, is surrounded by a wall full of receptor substances, we realize that this might be the worst trap of all. How would new virus particles ever get out of the cell where they were made, if they did not have this means of escape?

The interaction of virus and receptor substance has usually been looked at the other way around, that is, in connection with the entrance and not the exit of the virus particle. As long as only the entering virus particle was being studied, the situation appeared paradoxical; it seemed as though the virus, by automatically destroying the receptor substance which held it to the host cell, was literally sawing off the limb on which it sat. As a matter of fact the sawing-off process takes time; we have to assume that, before it is completed, further processes set in leading to infection of any cell which is a suitable host for the virus. In order to see what happens during and after infection we return to bacteriophages, where these processes have been most thoroughly studied and where they are best understood.

Experimental subdivision of the reproductive cycle: the infection of the host cell

Darkness (eclipse).—Micro-organisms multiply by dividing into two. It was long assumed that, once inside the cell, viruses follow the same multiplication scheme. Therefore the following observation, which was made in connection with several different types of virus, caused considerable surprise: If virus-infected cells are ground up at various intervals after infection, no active virus particles at all are found at first—not even those which were put in to infect the cells. According to expectation there should always be some viruses in the cell mash, and geometrically more, the more time that has passed since infection. Nothing of the kind could be observed. Though after some time active virus does again appear in the cell, between this point and the moment of infection there seemed to be a period of complete darkness. This period was dubbed "eclipse." It appeared very mysterious and some researchers tried to explain it away altogether. Today we recognize the eclipse as the crucial phase of virus-reproduction during which the synthesis of virus-nucleic acid and virus-protein, the two main components of the new particles, takes place. Most of the information on this subject has been gained from research with phage.

The infecting virus particle is destroyed.—Since phage particles adhere to the cell with the tips of their "tails" only, it seemed worthwhile to try to tear them off again simply by mechanical force and see what happened. In this way infection of the cell might be prevented, even though the first step in that direction, namely adsorption, had already been taken. It was assumed that the phage particle first attaches to the cell and then slips in. If step one could be experimentally separated from step two, both phases could be studied more easily.

The experiment had a curious result. It is true that if a bacterial suspension with adsorbed phage is vehemently stirred, some phage material is stripped off the cells. This material proves, however, to be not complete phages, but only their protein components. The nucleic acid component, on the other hand, remains with the cells, which go on to produce new phage particles, although they don't have at all a complete particle to use as a pattern.

This experiment killed two birds with one stone: it disposed of the assumption that viruses multiply by dividing in two ("binary fission") and it explained the strange "eclipse." Shortly after adsorption each phage particle is apparently carved up into its two main chemical components. One of these, the protein, is no longer necessary; the other, the nucleic acid, is taken up by the cell and there initiates the manufacture of new, complete phage particles. In the carving-up process the infecting particle loses its structural identity. This is why it cannot be found in the cell after infection.

The separation of the phage particle's component parts is confirmed by the electron microscope. Let us take another look at Figure 21, particularly the bacterium in the lower right corner of the photograph. The heads of nearly all the adsorbed phage particles appear strangely shrunken in comparison to the plump heads of the unattached particles. The same thing can be seen in Figure 20. Some of the phage particles which have reacted with free receptor substance are likewise sadly shrunken, so that one can just barely see their outlines. Chemical analysis proves that such a ghostly shade is nothing more nor less than the protein component of the phage particle. It still has the shape of the original particle but the nucleic acid strand or strands, which used to fill it, have slipped out.

The situation, then, is as follows: Shortly after the "tail" tip comes in contact with a host receptor, the phage nucleic acid slips over into the cell; only the empty protein "coat" remains outside, dangling uselessly from the cell wall, from which it may be stripped off without ill effect. In the meantime, phage nucleic acid and cell, together, form a new functional unit which goes to work immediately to make more phage particles. If the phage "tail" comes in contact with free receptor substance, the nucleic acid strands likewise slip out of the protein coat. In this case, of course, the nucleic acid is lost in the surrounding fluid and the phage particle as an infectious unit is finished.

We have now arrived at a new conception of the phage particle as a tiny hypodermic syringe filled with nucleic acid. Upon contact with a suitable receptor, the syringe automatically ejects its contents. Infection immediately follows adsorption. When we say the cell is infected, we mean it is ready and able to make new phage particles as soon as it has swallowed the nucleic acid of the adsorbed phage particle. The protein coat, on the other hand, has nothing to do with the actual reproduction of the virus; it merely serves as a protective covering for the sensitive nucleic acid, with the further function of delivering that nucleic acid to, and into, the cell. The nucleic acid would not be able to get in by itself; for this it requires the protein coat, and especially the "coat tail" containing the key which by chemical interactions unlocks the cell wall.

Just what happens when an animal virus infects a cell is not quite so well known. Some of these viruses also require a receptor substance as we have seen, and the eclipse is a phenomenon which has been found wherever it has been looked for, even among plant viruses. It can therefore safely be assumed that the infecting virus particle is always carved up immediately upon infection, which is why it is not to be found in the cell. A prerequisite for this is that the protein and nucleic acid components of the particle be easily separable. This has been shown to be the case for phages and can now also be proven for TMV. The rod-shaped particles of this latter virus (Fig. 15) are constructed like a candle: a nucleic acid strand is surrounded by a thick cylindrical coat of protein, just as the candlewick is surrounded by wax. Figure 22 shows such a rod-shaped particle from which some sections of the protein coat have been removed by chemical means, revealing the nucleic acid "wick." Incidentally, the nucleic acid strand (or strands)

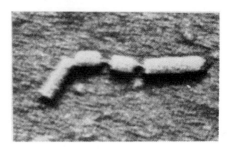

FIG. 22. The protein coat of this TMV particle has been removed in several places, revealing the nucleic acid strand which runs down the center. (G. Schramm, G. Schumacher, and W. Zillig, *Nature*, 175 [1955], 549.)

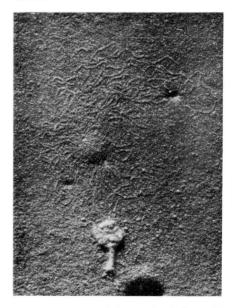

FIG. 23. An exploded particle of phage *T6*. The nucleic acid has been expelled and can be seen as a ball of matted strands next to the torn protein coat. Enlarged approximately 40,000 times. (D. Fraser and R. C. Williams, *Proc. Nat. Acad. Sci.*, 39 [1953], 750.)

of phage are much too long to lie stretched out in the particles; rather they are rolled up into a ball in the phage head. In Figure 23 we see a phage particle with an artificially exploded head. The ball of tangled nucleic acid thread has been expelled and can be distinguished lying next to the protein coat.

Plant viruses manage to get along without receptors in the plant cell wall, and without an entry key of their own. As we know, these viruses take advantage of accidental entries provided by boring and biting insects and other injuries to the plant. Since there is no receptor substance, the infecting particle is presumably not split up until after it has entered the cell. We may ask why no special infection mechanism, similar to that for phages and animal viruses, has developed here. For one thing, injuries to the plant are sufficiently common so that a specialized infection mechanism would be of no selective advantage to the plant virus. Perhaps such a mechanism even could not be developed, as the cellulose and other components of the plant cell wall are too inert and resistant to any attempts at hole-drilling by chemical means suited for including them in the outfit of a virus particle.

A puzzle.—The mechanism of phage infection which we have just described teaches an important lesson concerning self-replication. Previously (in Chapter III) speculations were based on the general idea that only structures composed of protein *and* nucleic acid are capable of autocatalytic reproduction. Since both chromosomes and viruses consist of these two substances, this was an obvious thought. The infection process of phages, however, reveals that in fact the nucleic acid alone is responsible for reproducing the whole particle. If an autocatalytic reproductive mechanism is involved at all, it can only apply to the nucleic acid. We can give up trying to construct models for self-reproducing proteins or indeed, entire virus particles.

Even though only the nucleic acid is taken from the infecting phage particle by the cell, the infected cell then goes on to make complete phage particles—protein bags filled with nucleic acid—and not just any odd type of phage, but the very type to which the infecting particle belonged. We know from our discussion of adsorption specificity that the fine structure of its protein is characteristic for each phage type. But since the protein part of the infecting particle never gets into the cell, it can never provide the pattern for the making of copies. Obviously the phage nucleic acid is the only source of pertinent "information" available to the cell. Therefore, the fine structure of the nucleic acid must be similarly specific and characteristic for each phage type, and the outstanding feature of this structure must be that the cell can "read" from it, as from a recipe, what kind of protein to make for the new generation of phage particles.

We now have a somewhat more detailed idea of how exact copies of viruses or similarly complex normal cell components are made. Protein synthesis and nucleic acid synthesis are interdependent indeed, but this interdependence is rather one-sided in a certain sense. Of the two, the nucleic acid alone is responsible for the hereditary continuity of both; it must symbolize recipes from which proteins can be made and it must also, in some way, serve as the pattern for its own exact reproduction.

Is it the nucleic acid, then, which, by multiplying autocatalytically, finally closes the biosynthetic cycle in autonomous cells? Possibly, yes. Whereas not much is yet known about the fine structure of RNA (Ribonucleic acid), some recent findings about the structure of DNA (Desoxyribonucleic acid) make a mechanism for its self-reproduction imaginable. DNA is the nucleic acid contained in phages and also in the genetic apparatus of cells.

The facts about DNA structure which had been ascertained by purely chemical means were given in Chapter III. Perhaps we should repeat them here: A DNA molecule is a long thread or chain consisting of thousands of links called nucleotides. There are four kinds of nucleotides which differ with respect to their base components. They can be arranged in any sequential order, whereby an enormous number of different DNA molecules can come into existence. So far it has not been possible to determine the exact sequence of these different nucleotides in any DNA strands. In this direction, then, the way to an absolute structural analysis of DNA is still blocked, which is most annoying.

Better progress has been made in another direction, namely, in answering the question whether DNA strands occur in the virus or cell nucleus singly or in bundles. They might be bundled without this being detectable by chemical means. It has now been established by means of X-ray crystallography and inspired model building that a certain type of bundling is indeed the rule. There are always two strands per bundle, which form a double helix by running parallel around an imaginary cylinder. It is easy to make a model of this structure: just take two wires and wind them parallelly round and round a wooden rod. Then remove the rod.

If you make the model, you will find that it is not at all easy to separate the two strands of the helix; they are interlocked once at each twist. However, this does not yet hold the DNA strands together as tightly as, according to measurements, they are actually held. The two strands are evidently fixed at a uniform distance from one another by additional forces. What are these forces? There is good reason to believe that the additional holding power is supplied by attraction between the base components of the two strands. The nucleotide bases are held together somewhat like magnets and thus form rigid ladder steps between the strands. We can now picture the whole structure as a sort of spiral staircase (Fig. 24). Its thickness is just above the visibility limits of the electron microscope (Fig. 23). The structural details can no

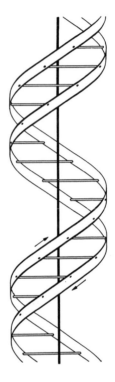

FIG. 24. Diagram of a section of the DNA double helix. At this magnification the entire molecule would be more than 200 yds. long. The two bands represent the nucleotide chains, and the paired bases are indicated by the cross bars. The vertical line shows the long axis of the spiral. (J. D. Watson and F. H. C. Crick, *Cold Spring Harbor Symp. Quant. Biol.*, 18 [1953], 123.)

longer be seen, but they can be deduced from indirect evidence.

There is a further point which is thought to clinch the argument for the double-strand structure as a duplicating mechanism. Each rung of the spiral staircase consists, as we said, of two bases, one from each of the DNA strands. At the point of contact the bases are held by mutual attraction, thus forming the rigid rungs. The four available bases are not of equal length, however; two of them are shorter and two are longer. Now, if the double helix is to be regular (as it is), then obviously no rung may consist of two long or two short bases; a short piece must always be connected to a long piece and then the distance between the two strands will remain constant, as it is actually found to be. The two short bases are Thymine (*T*) and Cytosine (*C*) and the longer ones are Adenine (*A*) and Guanine (*G*). Rungs of equal length could evidently be put together in four different ways, namely *A* and *T*, *A* and *C*, *G* and *T*, or *G* and *C*. However, a closer examination of the attractive forces among the respective bases reveals that, for physicochemical reasons, they are not very strong between *A* and *C*, and *G* and *T*. Consequently there are, after all, only two possible combinations, namely *A* and *T*, and *G* and *C*. Each rung must consist of one pair or the other of these.

If we think about these facts we come to a very important conclusion: Assuming that the sequence of nucleotides, as characterized by their bases, is known for one DNA strand, then it is immediately obvious what the only strand with which it can pair must look like. Let us write it down, minus the spiralization:

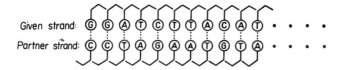

Given strand: G G A T C T T A C A T · · · ·
Partner strand: C C T A G A A T G T A · · · ·

The reader who has followed the discussion so far is now probably running ahead. He will guess how the structure we have been describing might go about making copies of itself. Let us assume the double spiral is opened up a bit at one end, so that the bases of the first rungs are torn apart like this:

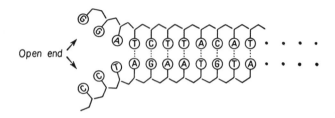

Instead of reuniting with each other, the separated strands might, by means of the specific attractive forces of their bases, pull appropriate nucleotides out of the environment. Each *A* would catch and hold a free *T*-nucleotide, each *T* an *A*, each *G* a *C*, and each *C* a *G:*

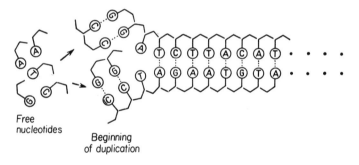

Here we have the beginnings of two double strands exactly like the first one. As more and more rungs of the original are torn apart—just like a zipper being opened—more bases are freed; each of these in turn grabs a new partner from among the free-floating nucleotides. By the time the process reaches the other end, two identical structures have been formed:

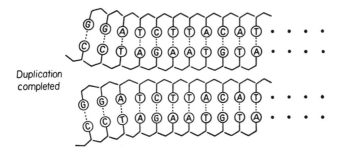

Duplication
completed

In each of the copies, one strand derives from the original sample and the other is newly constructed.

Since the whole process takes place inside a cell, the origin of the free nucleotides is no problem. The cell's chemical assembly lines can easily keep up a supply of the four types of nucleotides, so that the two new double strands can go on to repeat the reproductive process and produce four, which then make eight, and so forth, in typical autocatalytic fashion.

It all seems simple and crystal-clear, doesn't it? Unfortunately it must now be confessed that it is not certain whether nature actually uses this elegant method for DNA reproduction. I hope the reader has gotten some fun out of playing the chemical puzzle game for its own sake. Certainly he has learned something about the thoughts of those who are engaged in biochemical research today. The most successful research derives from the ability to build bold theoretical constructions on a foundation of known fact. The testing of such a hypothesis then leads to the framing of new questions, the discovery of further facts, and an increase in understanding. A theory as clearly formulated as the one about DNA reproduction is more valuable for research than a new apparatus for the laboratory. It leads to new experiments which would not otherwise have been thought of, and which will have interesting results, whether they prove the theory or not.

To repeat briefly, the idea is this: In certain viruses, and possibly in all true living organisms, the sole carrier of hereditary "information" is a chemical substance called DNA. It guarantees identity between parents and progeny. Consequently, some mechanism must exist for making exact copies of this DNA. A mechanism of this sort, very plausible at first sight, could be derived from the structure of the DNA molecule itself! On closer examination, though, the postulated mechanism needs some modification, at least, even if accepted as basically correct. But we need not go into that here. Suffice it to say that difficulties arise from the spiralization which does not permit the partner strands to separate so easily.

Writing in code.—Not only does the DNA have to duplicate itself, it must also bring about the production of specific proteins. For instance, under the direction of phage DNA, protein coats for phage particles have to be manufactured, and these must have, not only a specific fine structure, but also a characteristic total shape. When we learned that only the DNA portion of the infecting particle enters the cell, we already concluded that this DNA must contain a recipe for the preparation of complete phage particles. How does the structure of the DNA molecule provide for preserving written information?

The answer to this question can be seen in the picture of a DNA strand which we drew up. The four types of nucleotides can be used to construct a vast number of code words. It has to be pointed out that here we are considering only one of the two strands in the DNA double helix and that, therefore, the sequence of nucleotides is not governed by any rule. (The fact that the order of nucleotides in one strand determines a complementary order in the partner strand is significant for the duplicating mechanism but not for our present discussion.) Thus, if we could "read" the strand and one section of it said, "*AT-AGAGCGTACCTACTTCCG*," then this might mean, for the cell: "Link such-and-such amino acids (protein building blocks) together to make a piece of phage coat." The sequence, *"CACTAAATCGGTCTGT"* might spell out quite a different combination of amino acids such as would be required to make a certain enzyme molecule, and so forth. The possibilities for passing on written information with this system are enormous. It almost seems extravagant of nature to have provided four symbols where two would do; as we all know the Morse code contains only the dot and the dash, and yet with these two symbols anything from stock quotations to lyrical poetry can be transmitted.

The Morse code represents the twenty-six letters of the alphabet by combination of two symbols, whereas the nucleotide code has to provide for at least thirty letters—that is to say, approximately thirty different amino acids—from combinations of four symbols. In both cases symbols of a higher order are formed by combining the letters, into words and sentences in the case of the Morse code, and into amino acid sequences or whole protein molecules in the case of the nucleotide alphabet.

We can extend the comparison: the DNA double-helix which the phage particle sends into the cell is like the paper strip, covered with dots and dashes, which comes out of the telegraph machine. In both cases a long strip of material is used to transmit coded messages to a recipient who understands the code.

The nucleotide code is understood by the cell but not by the scientist. He is in the position of someone who looks over the telegraph operator's shoulder wishing to decipher the message, but who does not know the Morse code. Of course one could spend a lot of time observing the sequence of dots and dashes and seeing how the telegraph operator responds to them. In this way one might eventually learn the meaning of the symbols and perhaps even reconstruct the Morse alphabet. There are, however, modern code-breaking methods which would be more efficient.

Actually the scientist's position is even worse. Neither of these approaches can be used for deciphering the nucleotide alphabet because as yet there is no way of determining the nucleotide sequence in a given DNA strand. We mentioned this earlier, and now the reader will understand why we spoke of it as "most annoying." As long as not even the symbol sequence of a code can be determined, it is of course impossible to understand the relationship between symbol combinations and the responses to them. It is as if the telegraph operator nastily kept us from getting a good look at the code strip. All we know is that the message contains intelligible directions, because, after studying them, the operator takes certain deliberate actions. But from this we can only draw the general inference that the sequence of symbols on the strip (respectively, the sequence of nucleotides in the DNA strand) is not random; it must represent a system of writing.

The determination of DNA nucleotide sequence is a purely chemical problem which will presumably be solved soon. The next step will be to learn the "alphabet" of this language—that is, to translate the four nucleotide symbols into the thirty amino acid "letters." After this it might become possible to "read" the message on a DNA strand. Finally, and far in the future, a whole DNA archive as it is contained in the genes of every cell might become accessible to the researcher. It seems more likely now than ever that the genes are DNA molecules or rather parts thereof, and we can begin to understand how they function. A set of genes determines the cell's chemical possibilities by permitting only certain protein molecules to be formed; these in turn, as enzymes for instance, mediate specific chemical assembly lines. Knowing something about DNA reproduction, we can also understand how each daughter cell gets an exact copy of each gene and thus inherits the same chemical capabilities from the mother cell.

Mutation.—We can even understand how mutations come about. You will remember that we defined a mutation as a hereditary change in an assembly line system. Everybody makes mistakes, and the mechanisms of viruses are no exception. If a mistake is made while the genes are being copied, however, and one of the daughter cells gets a DNA strand in which the nucleotide sequence differs from that in the mother cell, then the consequences may be serious. The message on the incorrect copy will have changed in meaning, or perhaps it will be meaningless. The old family recipe for making a certain protein, for example an enzyme, is lost and the hapless daughter has to follow a new recipe and make something else, which will probably be useless, or nothing at all if the garbled copy is entirely unintelligible. In either case the result will be that a certain assembly line will lack a certain worker, namely the enzyme with its special structure and function. The work on that line will be disturbed, probably stopped, and the normal chemical end product will not be turned out.

Depending on which assembly lines it happens to hit, this mutation mechanism can evoke the most varied peculiarities among living organisms. In the discussion of receptor substances we examined one such mutation, which even proved useful for the cell. Quite often, on the other hand, the mutation disrupts an assembly line whose proper functioning is vital to the cell. In this event, of course, the cell cannot continue to live, but is doomed to death (such a mutation is called a lethal mutation) unless the biochemist comes to the rescue. Under certain circumstances he is able to do this—for example, if he can find out which vital substance the cell is no longer able to make. If he supplies the missing substance, and the cell is able to take it in, the situation is saved. The cell continues to live and to produce offspring.

Of course the offspring can likewise be kept alive only if they are supplied with the missing substance, because the defective gene-copy from the mother cell is always copied now in this changed form. Even if, in a later generation, another mistake is made, and the nucleotide sequence is changed again, it is highly unlikely that, of the infinite possible arrangements of the nucleotides, just the original one should be reconstructed. Of course it is not impossible, but we must remind ourselves again and again that these processes are running on blindly, without purpose or afterthought. There is no factor or force known to us which could intervene here and make the unlikely even a tiny bit more likely.

The chemical forces which tend to keep things going normally are very powerful and the chances for an irregularity to crop up at all are small indeed; for most genes only one copy in 100 million is defective. This ratio, which can be determined experimentally and quite accurately for any identifiable gene, is called the "mutation rate." This normally very low mutation rate can be artificially increased by means of irradiation with harmful rays of various kinds (such as are produced by atom bomb explosions). Certain chemicals also increase the rate of spontaneous mutation. Increasing the mutation rate only means that some disturbing accidents are given a better chance to arise. Exactly what happens remains accidental. No matter how the organism is treated, there is no certain way to evoke a particular gene mutation and thus make an accident into a rule.

It is easy to see why this should be so. The specificity of DNA molecules resides in the specific sequential arrangement of their component nucleotides. Yet so far, only a cell's delicate biochemical machinery knows how to discriminate between one sequence, i. e., one DNA molecule, and another. For our own clumsy chemicals or rays, DNA is just DNA—no matter what the sequence is. With such coarse means we can hit DNA all right, but with them we will never be able to aim our hits, which would be necessary to produce desired and predictable effects.

By employing the principle of the nucleotide code, nature has most shrewdly protected herself from "creative" whims of man. Or else there would be no end of composing artificial supermen or other monsters in biochemical laboratories. Strangely enough, some biochemists seem to regret the dim prospects of ever achieving this.

The above considerations apply to viruses as well as to genes in cells. A mistake in copying a virus DNA strand results in a mutation. Since a change in the DNA fine structure automatically changes the corresponding protein, which, in this case, is the protein coat of the virus particle, the effects may be very dramatic. Take a phage particle, for instance, whose "tail" tip determines which cell-receptors the particle can adhere to; you can imagine the consequences of a mutation affecting the DNA recipe for this "tail" tip protein. It may mean that the phage particle can no longer enter a certain host cell, or, on the other hand, that it can now get into cells which were taboo for its ancestors.

The latter type of phage mutants are easy to find, isolate and grow: a large number of phage particles are spread on a lawn of bacteria which are ordinarily resistant to the phage type being applied. None of the normal phage particles will therefore be able to produce plaques. If any plaques *are* found under these conditions, they must come from mutant phages with a changed—that is to say, enlarged—host range. It is an easy matter to remove some particles from such a colony of mutants and grow them separately. The stock of mutant phages is then available for further experiments and comparisons with the ancestral strain.

The extreme case of the lethal mutation also exists among viruses. For example, the nucleotide sequence of a mutated particle may be so scrambled that no host cell is able to make head or tail of the message. In that event the mutant virus cannot direct the production of offspring; it must remain the only representative of its decadent kind. Not even the biochemist can save it because viruses have no chemical assembly lines which could be supplied with missing intermediary products.

Experimental subdivision of the reproductive cycle: the host cell makes new virus particles

We now return to the main theme of this chapter, the reproductive cycle of the virus particle. We had reached the point in the story where the host cell has just "swallowed" the DNA double-spiral of a virus particle. Next we would like to know about the production of new virus-nucleic acid and virus-protein by the infected cell: what raw materials are these substances derived from, in what quantities, in what order are they synthesized, and at what point does their combination into new virus particles begin?

Also we would like to have some experimental proof that the DNA spiral actually multiplies geometrically (1-2-4-8-16, and so forth). In the phage-infected bacterial cell this would mean that the DNA double-spiral from the infecting phage particle must have the same fate as all of its daughter spirals. They all must keep on duplicating over and over again, as long as they have time, and their time is not up until, one by one, they are packed into protein "tail" coats and sent out of the exploded host cell as new phage particles. Actually we shall see that the fate of the infecting DNA strand, or at least our knowledge about it, is very dim.

Raw materials.—If the bacterial cells were "eaten" by the phages, then all the matter—that is to say, all the atoms—which goes to make up a new phage generation would have to come directly from the host cell. This is really quite obvious; if a lioness has, from the time of her birth, been fed exclusively on lamb, then her cubs can only contain atoms which were originally lamb atoms. We will not go into the reorganization which is necessary to change lamb meat into lion meat.

We already know that phages do not eat bacteria in the ordinary sense. Since the mass of new phage particles produced by an infected cell represents only a fraction of the total cell mass, however, it is still possible that some of the cell material is simply chopped up into amino acids and nucleotides and then converted into virus material.

At this point we recall that an infected cell only makes new viruses in the presence of nutrients. Of course energy is needed if simple building-block molecules are to be assembled into complex structures, and so we could imagine that virus-infected cells use the nutrients exclusively as a source of energy for the forced labor of making new viruses. In that case the new virus particles would contain energy but not matter derived from the nutrients. On the other hand it is also possible that virus-infected cells use nutrients in two ways, just as noninfected cells do—as a source of energy as well as for the construction of certain materials which can be used to make new virus particles. In this case the new viruses would have to contain atoms that came from the nutrients which the cell took in after infection.

Is there any way to find out which of these possibilities is actually correct? What would be needed is a means of marking atoms so that they could be spotted in any molecule combination they may enter. In this way all possible sources of virus raw material could be tagged to determine precisely the answer to our question. Atoms can, in fact, be marked by being made radioactive. Radioactive phosphorus atoms, for example, behave just like ordinary phosphorus atoms except that a certain fraction of them explodes in any given period of time, thereby emitting rays which can be measured.

Now suppose one wants to determine the source of the phosphorus in phage DNA. The phosphorus-containing nutrients which are supplied to the infected cell are marked with radioactive phosphorus. The amount of radioactivity in the virus particles released from the cells is then measured. Any radioactive phosphorus found here must derive from nutrients the cell took in after infection; the remaining phosphorus atoms must have belonged to the cell before infection. The exact proportions can be calculated, or, if the experiment is done the other way around, measured directly. Bacterial cells are then fed on radioactive phosphorus until they are quite full; next they are infected with phage and, at the same time, the radioactive nutrients are replaced by nutrients containing ordinary phosphorus. Any radioactive phosphorus which is now found in the newly made phage particles must have been taken in by the cell, for its own use, before infection.

Radioactive atoms used in this way are called "tracers." From the tracer experiments described above we learn that more than three-fourths of the total phosphorus in a new crop of phages comes from nutrients which the cell took in after infection; the remainder is contributed by the cell from its own stores. Corresponding experiments with nitrogen and carbon tracers yield approximately the same results.

If we did not know it before, we certainly know now that the virus-infected cell is not simply a passive victim —it does more than merely contribute its own material for conversion into virus material. While a small part of cell matter is converted in this way, the main function of the cell is to do what it has always done—to take up nutrients and change them into energy and building blocks by means of its chemical assembly lines. In the virus-infected cell, however, these products no longer serve the needs of the cell itself but are used exclusively to make new virus particles.

This complete switch in the productive mechanism of the cell is evidently commanded by the DNA from the infecting virus particle. For some reason, which is ·not yet understood, this DNA has more power over the cell than its own DNA—which is simply not listened to any more.

The existing assembly lines, however, are preserved for the time being. But the enzyme molecules which serve these assembly lines can no longer be replaced; they keep the chemical turnover going for a while and produce virus particles as long as they can. Eventually the enzymes are worn out and suddenly the whole system breaks down. The cell becomes defective and bursts, hurling out the virus particles completed up to then together with the debris of the formerly highly organized system.

A complete breakdown—and why? Because the cell has not been producing enzymes and other things which are needed to keep the chemical cycle going. Instead the bacterial cell was forced to produce virus particles which misfit this cycle because they contribute nothing to it. They are a costly end product since they are completely useless from the cell's point of view. At the moment when the DNA from the infecting virus particle pushed aside the bacterial DNA, which was responsible for the continuity of the cycle ("life"), that cycle was opened and became, instead, a dead-end street. The cell was doomed to death at the moment of infection, but, interestingly enough, it continued to operate its chemical assembly lines for a while as though nothing had happened.

In this situation the cell is really like a test tube in which just the right enzymes and other needed substances are brought together with some simple raw materials (sugar, ammonia, phosphoric acid) for the synthesis of a single product—virus. The contents of the test tube can only perform this one feat; they cannot regenerate themselves, which would mean producing more test tubes with more contents. The whole process has a beginning and an end and is, in this sense, quite similar to those feats which the chemist can already perform in the laboratory when he combines certain chemicals and has them synthesize a particular substance. Between this type of synthesis in vitro and the synthesis of viruses in the cell there is a difference in complexity but not in kind. Once all the mate rials which must interact during virus synthesis are known, it will be possible to make viruses in a test tube just as starch granules, for example, are synthesized in the laboratory today. Twenty years ago nobody would have believed that to be possible either.

Let us continue our discussion of the materials involved in virus synthesis. The use of tracers makes it possible to find out what kind of its own material the cell sacrifices to make virus particles. It turns out to be primarily *its own DNA!* Of course the bacterial DNA is no longer of any use to the cell anyway and might as well be utilized for something else. Scientifically speaking, however, this is a very sloppy and unconvincing argument. It would really be important to know what forces the bacterial DNA to become mere raw material for virus DNA. The turnover could occur through breakdown into nucleotides which then would form completely unspecific building blocks for the duplication of the virus DNA. Or else—as is also conceivable—chunks of bacterial DNA, including some whole code words, could be taken over by the virus. Suppose these code words, as expressed by a certain nucleotide sequence, are already found in the virus DNA anyway (either accidentally, or because of an evolutionary relationship between virus and bacterium); in that case the taking over of chunks of bacterial DNA by the virus would have no noticeable effect, except perhaps to shorten the virus duplication process very slightly because most of the virus DNA has to be nearly synthesized anyway by the infected cell. If, on the other hand, typically bacterial code words, foreign to the virus, were taken over into the virus DNA, then among the virus progeny a few particles would be produced which differ from the infecting parent particle. This sort of thing is actually found under certain conditions, but as a rule the bacterial code seems to be erased and the strands broken down into unspecific (nucleotide) form during DNA transfer. Here we have stumbled on the interesting problem of a possible hereditary relationship between bacteria and viruses, which, in turn, relates to the question of how viruses arose in the first place. More about this later in Chapter VIII.

Unlike bacterial DNA, bacterial protein seems to be of hardly any use for virus synthesis. The cell must start from scratch to make the protein coats for the new virus particles. For this, of course, it uses the nutrients which are taken up after infection. Again a superficial explanation comes to mind: if the cell proteins were cleaned up like the cell DNA, the assembly lines, which are needed for virus synthesis, would very soon stop running for lack of enzymes, which, after all, are proteins. Here, too, chemical forces are involved which are not understood yet and which really determine that the bacterial DNA be used up and the bacterial protein be left alone. Utility is never a determining factor in such processes.

Intermediate product: nucleic acid.—We now turn to the intermediate products of virus synthesis. Fortunately there are some phages with a type of DNA which differs slightly in its chemical make-up from that of the host cell. This makes it possible to determine at any time after infection how much of its own DNA the cell still contains and how much virus DNA is now present. At various intervals, infected cells are artificially broken open; all the DNA is then extracted and separated, by chemical means. into bacterial and virus DNA. In this way DNA conversion as well as net synthesis of virus DNA from the moment of infection to the lysis of the cell can be plotted on a curve.

Such a curve shows that, after a short pause of a few minutes, subsequent to infection, the cell begins to fill up with virus DNA, and at the same time to lose its own DNA. In view of our discussion above this is not surprising; we already know about the conversion of cell DNA into virus DNA. It is interesting to know, however, how much virus DNA is produced per time-unit, for instance per minute. Our first thought would be that the increase is not constant but grows from minute to minute—assuming that the DNA strands really multiply according to our model, that is, geometrically. If, on the other hand, the reproductive mechanism is not based on division, then the increase would have to be constant, that is, during each minute the came quantity of virus DNA would have to be added to the amount already on hand (arithmetic increase).

Is this the crucial experiment which is going to determine once and for all whether we are dealing with an autocatalytic template mechanism or not? It becomes doubtful when we consider that a chain is only as strong at its weakest link. No factory can produce faster than the supply of raw materials permits. If a bottleneck develops in the delivery of raw materials, it does not matter how big the manufacturing plant is—the turnout of finished products cannot be speeded up. End products leave the factory at the same rate at which the raw material which is the most difficult to procure can be supplied. Similarly the fastest tempo of DNA synthesis must be determined by the speed at which the cell's assembly lines can turn out new nucleotides. Assembly lines, however, produce arithmetically, not geometrically. Thus, even if a constant doubling of all existing DNA strands in true geometric fashion resulted in more and more machinery for the conversion of nucleotides into DNA, this wouldn't necessarily show up on the curve. Since each time the total number of conversion machines (DNA strands) is doubled, each of them receives only half as much raw material per time-unit as before (after another doubling, one quarter, and so forth), it now takes twice as long (four times as long, and so forth) until the total number can again be doubled. What it all adds up to is that the total DNA increases by the same amount each minute.

This is just what the curve shows; the total amount of virus DNA produced in the cell increases in proportion to the time elapsed, so that it is not possible to draw any conclusions about the type of reproductive mechanism involved. Either a geometric (autocatalytic) mechanism, or an arithmetic (stamp or assembly line) mechanism fits the experimental results, since we can be sure that the cell cannot constantly increase its rate of nucleotide production.

It should be added that the production curves for geometric and arithmetic reproductive mechanisms do not have to look exactly the same, even if the supply of raw material is limited. The two curves only begin to coincide when this limit of supply is reached, assuming there was an excess to begin with. An assembly line (an arithmetic mechanism) pays no attention to oversupply; it keeps right on working at an even tempo. A geometric mechanism, on the other hand, if it is supplied with an excess of raw material, works faster and faster, until supply and output are evenly balanced. A geometric production curve will, under these conditions, rise steeply at first, and only straighten out when the balance point is reached, whereas an arithmetic curve will rise in a straight line right from the start. Consequently a very careful analysis of the first part of the curve might, after all, give some clue as to the type of reproductive mechanism involved. Of course there would have to be an initial excess of free nucleotides in the cell. About this, however, nothing definite is as yet known, and, furthermore the present analytical techniques are probably not precise enough to reveal a short bend in the beginning of the curve, even if it does exist. Anyhow it hasn't been found, and so experimental evidence for one or the other reproductive mechanism is still lacking.

The curve showing DNA balance answers some other questions, though: How long does the linear increase of virus DNA in the cell continue, and when do new, complete virus particles begin to appear, thus ending the period of eclipse? The answer to both questions is clear-cut. The amount of virus DNA keeps on increasing in the infected cell until it bursts. The first complete virus particles, however, appear in the cell much earlier, about ten minutes after infection, a long time before lysis. The cells have to be artificially opened then so that any completed phage particles can be extracted and their presence demonstrated by means of the plaque test. It is most convenient to run a series of plaque tests simultaneously with the recording of the DNA balance curve. Then the total amount of virus DNA found at any one time can be subdivided into that which is already packed into new virus particles and a further quantity which is still unpackaged.

It turns out that by the tenth minute after infection enough virus DNA has accumulated to equip about 40–80 phage particles. After the tenth minute we do not suddenly find 40–80 new phage particles, however; these appear in an orderly fashion, one after the other. They increase arithmetically and at approximately the same rate as the amount of total virus DNA. This means that there is always a surplus of DNA equal to that which had accumulated up to the tenth minute.

This excess would not be especially interesting if it merely represented some kind of side-product, maybe an imperfect sort of DNA made only during the first ten minutes, which somehow cannot be used to make virus particles. Another possibility—much more exciting and now proven in fact—is that the surplus represents a sort of intracellular virus DNA "pool." On one side it "rains" into the pool, whereas from the other side the pool keeps on being drained, so that it neither runs over nor dries out, but always remains at the same level. Stated more precisely this means that the pool consists of an accumulation of virus DNA helices. Nucleotides keep raining in and are used for the duplication of the DNA strands. Simultaneously and at the same rate, complete helices are removed and packed into protein coats to make new phage particles. The pool arises because the packaging mechanism does not begin to function until ten minutes after infection; the first newly made DNA helices are thus not immediately used but have a chance to accumulate.

The packaging mechanism is of particular interest relative to the question of geometric vs. arithmetic duplication. Here we have one partial mechanism of virus synthesis which most certainly operates like an assembly line, that is, arithmetically. The newly completed phage particles leave this assembly line one after the other, as is proven by their arithmetic increase. The techniques for detecting individual virus particles are precise enough to establish that. If there is geometric duplication involved in virus synthesis, it could only take place in the aforementioned DNA pool.

Intermediate product: protein.—The second intermediate product of virus synthesis is the protein for particle coats. Whereas all aspects of DNA production are beyond the visibility limits of even the electron microscope and can thus only be analyzed indirectly, we can get a tiny glimpse at protein coat production. The most important happenings, of course, are invisible here too.

If phage-infected cells are broken open at regular intervals after infection, and their contents examined under the electron microscope, nothing special is found at first —nothing, that is, except the various tiny granules and sticky masses of protoplasm which one would expect. Infected cells which are not opened until nine minutes after infection, however, suddenly show some roundish empty structures which look like phage heads. Rodlike structures which might be precursors of phage "tails" are also found (Fig. 25). With serological and other methods it can be proven that these two structures actually consist of the same chemical material as the corresponding parts of the phage coat. The head and "tail" are usually not joined at this time; if they are, it is so loose a connection that they are torn apart when the cell is opened. Nor is the head covering characteristically filled with DNA; if so, it slips out easily for lack of a "stopper." It seems reasonable to

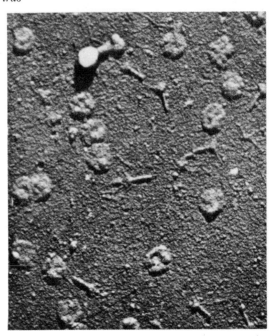

FIG. 25. Components of incomplete phage particles. The flat, roundish structures consist of the same protein as the covering of finished phage particles but are not filled with nucleic acid (compare the single complete phage particle at the top left). Short rods, which are parts of phage "tails," can also be distinguished. (E. Kellenberger, Geneva.)

assume that these empty structures are unripe phage particles which have been from their "mother's womb untimely ripp'd." Indeed if the brutal deed is delayed just one minute longer, until the tenth minute, then one finds, in addition to the "unripe" structures, the first complete phage particles: head and "tail" here stick together and the head is stuffed full of DNA. They are infectious, too, as expected—we have already noted that the first infectious particles appear around the tenth minute—whereas the "unripe" forms are incapable of infecting a cell or producing any sort of offspring.

Instead of solving problems, the finding of these empty phage coats seems to complicate matters. How, for example, is the DNA to get out of the pool and into the heads? If the DNA helices are really reproducing autocatalytically in the pool, they must be lying there rather loosely—certainly not so tightly packed as in the phage heads. Each helix is, furthermore, extremely long, much longer than the entire bacterial cell, assuming that the total DNA of a phage particle is contained in only one double helix. Under these conditions the imagined pool of at least 40-80 double helices turns into a rather horribly messy spaghetti heap. How are we to conceive of a mechanism which reaches into this heap, grabs a helix which happens not to be involved in reproduction just then, rolls it up tightly, and hastily packs it into an empty head? One may be tempted to abandon the concept of an autocatalytic reproductive mechanism right at this point in favor of a stamp or assembly line mechanism for DNA reproduction. The messy spaghetti heap is then avoided and the whole process may be made to seem a bit more orderly. But this is not a sufficient reason to do so, and anyway the problem of how the long strands are to be rolled up into tight little packets still remains. Perhaps, instead of the pack of strands being stuffed into the finished protein cover, it happens the other way around, and the cover is woven on the surface of the DNA packet out of amino acids or larger building blocks. This possibility seems to be supported by certain experimental results which indicate that the DNA of a prospective phage particle is always finished before its protein coat.

Finished product.—Having examined the virus reproductive cycle in detail we now arrive at the end product. If everything has gone according to plan, the new particles will be exactly like the parent particle which sacrificed itself in order to bring children into the world in an involved sort of way. Involved though this method of reproduction may seem, it is still, in a sense, the simplest system in nature. Imagine the chemical mechanisms which must be set in motion to produce not just a few simple virus particles but whole cells, not to speak of multicellular organisms such as plants and animals!

Virus reproduction does not always follow the "normal" course. We have discussed the accidental and rare occurrences of mutations which result in offspring that differ from the parent particles; we also mentioned that the occasional exchange of "code words" (hereditary factors) between virus and host cell may have a similar effect. Even stranger things may happen along these lines. For example, given the chance, viruses in the reproductive phase may carry on a rather extensive love life among themselves, which also can result in new types being produced. In still other cases viruses may enter into so intimate and lengthy a relationship with the host cell that one can think of it as a sort of marriage.

Before we go on to discuss these subjects in more detail, such facts as are known about the reproductive cycle of virus types other than phage should be given. Compared to bacteriophage other viruses are not so well understood. This is not due to a lack of effort, but to various technical problems which make it particularly difficult to draw conclusions about events in the individual infected cell from mass experimental data. Just this is necessary, however, if biochemical mechanisms are to be uncovered. So long as only mass phenomena can be studied, their analysis, which is necessarily statistical, may obsure important clues.

No technique has yet been developed, for instance, for infecting a known number of plant cells with viruses, nor can the virus particles themselves be accurately counted. Nevertheless, it has recently been established in the case of tobacco mosaic virus that the nucleic acid portion of the particle, RNA in this case, is also infectious by itself. In other words the protein component is not involved in the transfer of genetic information here either, which

proves again that the nucleic acids (DNA as well as RNA)
are the sole carriers of heredity. When and where, during
the normal process of infection, the plant virus particle is
split into its component parts is not known.

One would also like to find out in what form the virus infection spreads throughout the plant. Must the entire reproductive cycle, up to and including the completion of
new particles, be run through in the cell which was originally infected, and are these new particles then carried
into neighboring cells by plasma streams? Or alternatively,
can the infection be spread inside the plant by some kind
of intermediate stages, for instance naked nucleic acid
strands or even some sort of die-stamp machines for making them? The answers to these very interesting questions
would provide much information about reproductive
mechanisms in general. Unfortunately, many technical
difficulties so far prevent us from making use of the special construction of plants with their interconnected cell
system which in principle would be so useful to answer
just those questions.

Mutations also occur among plant viruses. Mutated particles no longer produce the same disease symptoms in the
plant as the parent type. This is how the mutants are recognized, and they can then be isolated and grown separately. No doubt a change in the disease symptoms is due
to a change in the fine structure of the virus particle.
Sometimes detailed examination of the mutant virus protein reveals such a structural change. It is, of course, not
yet absolutely known that such structural changes in the
protein result from corresponding changes in the nucleic
acid, but it is definitely to be assumed.

Many plant viruses, and especially TMV, seem to have
a simple and regular type of protein which may turn out
to be very suitable for studying the structural correspond-
ence with nucleic acid. Thus perhaps the first attempts
at translating from nucleic acid language to protein language or vice versa will be made with plant viruses.

The various phases of the plant virus reproductive cycle have not been clearly distinguished. However, as with bacteriophage, "unripe" forms of these viruses are found in the extract of cells which have also produced complete viruses. It is not certain that these nucleic acid-free structures were on their way to being filled with nucleic acid and becoming virus particles; they might represent some kind of side product of virus synthesis. (This possibility has not been entirely excluded for the "unripe" phages either.) If more were known about this, more could be said about how nucleic acid and protein get together to form the complete virus particle. Are the two parts made by independent branches of the production system and then assembled, or is one part constructed like a mosaic on/in the other? The same problems crop up everywhere and it is not even guaranteed that they are always solved in the same way; what is valid for RNA-containing viruses, for instance, may not always apply to those which contain DNA.

"Incomplete" forms are also found among animal- and human-pathogenic viruses, sometimes even as the main product of a synthesis which has somehow gone haywire. These structures are of special interest because they can be compared with artificial breakdown products of complete virus particles in order to study the sometimes complicated anatomy of the latter. It seems that many animal viruses have a complicated construction of several different layers. It is not surprising to find that the outermost layer is attracted to the receptor substances of the cell; it enables the entire particle to attach to the host cell, there to pursue its evil designs. If this outer layer is removed, something remains which still holds all the nucleic acid (RNA) of the particle, but is no longer infectious, presumably because it is now unable to attach to the cell. Whether in the normal course of infection only this inner portion or even less of the particle gets into the cell, or whether the whole particle enters, is not known. Certainly

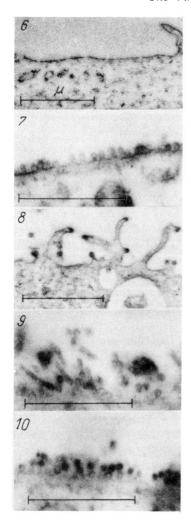

FIG. 26. Consecutive stages of virus production by cells of the chorioallantoic membrane (compare Fig. 4). (G. Hotz and W. Schäfer, Z. *Naturforschg.,* 10*b* [1955], 1.)

the nucleic acid, RNA again, enters the cell, and recently it could be demonstrated, as in the case of TMV, that nothing else is needed to instigate virus reproduction. It seems to push right up into the nucleus where it starts giving orders.

The reproductive cycle of these animal viruses takes several hours. At the end, the host cells do not burst, but secrete newly made virus particles for some time. This can be seen very clearly with the help of the electron microscope. During the period of eclipse, that is, so long as the cell contains no complete virus, nothing special can be observed under the electron microscope. Suddenly, however, the outside wall of the cell begins to show an eruption of blisters which rapidly increase in numbers (Fig. 26). At the same time the blisters begin to fill up with matter until they contain proper virus particles. These now free themselves from each other and from the host cell, probably by means of a built-in enzyme. From then on there is nothing to prevent the newly made viruses from attaching to other cells and producing a host of offspring until every available and suitable cell is destroyed. By this time, if the virus is one of the cold viruses and the host is you, you have certainly got a nasty cold with sore throat and bronchitis.

It is interesting that new particles are not observed deeper inside the host cell. The component parts seem to be manufactured nearer the middle of the cell, but they are too small to be seen directly. Their final assembly, anyway, appears to take place in the outer layer. What makes the inside of the cell wall the chosen place for this? Such stepwise construction at different localities is a bit difficult to reconcile with the anarchy which would have to reign in a nucleic acid pool as discussed earlier.

v. *The Love Life of Viruses*

So far we have been dealing with the "normal" reproductive cycle which results in a new generation of viruses
exactly like the parent. The continuity from generation to
generation is preserved by the nucleic acid. Occasional
spontaneous changes in the structure of the nucleic acid
result in offspring which differ from the parent, and these
changes are called mutations. Such mutations are not
based on any laws but are due to chance.

There are, however, other changes which follow certain
definite laws and thus have nothing to do with mutations.
It is perfectly well known that children are not exactly
like their parents, not because they are mutants but because they contain combinations from the hereditary material of both their parents. The mixing of parental hereditary factors or genes takes place according to certain
laws, known as Mendelian laws. Among viruses of course,
there is nothing to mix in the "normal" case where only
one virus particle, or even several of the same type, enter
the cell.

Recombination

What happens, however, if one host cell is infected by
two particles which are not exactly identical? Does the
cell get confused and, for lack of clear directives, produce
nothing? Or does it make freaks? Not at all. Let us take
the simplest case and look at the result. Bacterial cells are
simultaneously infected with phage particles which have
different host ranges; for one of these phage types, the
"normal" type, certain strains of bacteria are taboo,
whereas the other phage, which arose from the normal by
mutation, can enter such bacteria, thanks to its changed
DNA (protein) structure. We find that the cell which was
simultaneously infected with these two phage types reproduces the two types side by side. There is no confusion. The two different DNA structures are copied independently, which fits in with the model for autocatalytic
DNA reproduction. According to this model the cell's job
is the unspecific one of supplying nucleotides, which the
two DNA helices then use, each according to its own structure, to duplicate themselves. When a new virus particle
is put together it receives one or the other sort of DNA,
and accordingly it possesses, and passes on, the narrower
or the wider host range. So far there is no evidence of mixing. The DNA of each infecting particle seems to be
treated as a unit during reproduction; normal DNA remains normal DNA and mutant DNA remains mutant
DNA.

Let us go a step further. Another mutant which can be
isolated from the normal phage type has the same host
range as the normal but produces a bigger plaque on the
test plate. This characteristic is hereditary and, of course,
immediately recognizable; such a big plaque shows up
very clearly even among a large number of normal small
plaques. A culture of phages from the large plaque proved
to produce the large plaques consistently on all subse-

quent test plates. Thus a new mutant stock had been isolated for use in further experiments.

Now, for the mixture experiment. The question is: What kind of particles does the cell produce if it is infected with one of each of the mutant phage types? To repeat once more, one of the parent types makes small plaques like the normal type, but has a wider host range, whereas the other parent has the same narrow host range as the normal but makes large plaques. The result of this experiment is that the doubly infected host cell makes the two particle types side by side as in the previous experiment. But in addition two further phage types with which the host cell never came in contact are produced this time: One type is in every respect normal (small plaques, narrow host range) and another type combines the mutant characteristics of both parents (large plaques, wide host range). These particles, which differ from the parent types, occur with such frequency and regularity that there can be no question of mutation as a cause. Anyway it is obvious that we are dealing with a mixture effect. We can see that very clearly if we write symbols for the various characters:

> small plaques: *sm*   narrow host range: *n*
> large plaques: *lg*   wide host range: *w*

The experiment is then written like this:

> parents: *sm/w* and *lg/n*
> offspring: *sm/w* and *lg/n*
> plus: *sm/n* and *lg/w*
> ("normal") ("double mutant")

Among the offspring all four possible combinations are represented. Two of them owe their existence to an exchange, or recombination, of the parental traits and are therefore called "recombinants." The recombinants can be grown separately and will pass on the new combination of characters to their descendants.

The recombination of characters can also happen the other way around. In another experiment the recombinants are used as the parents for the double infection of a bacterial cell:

> parents: *sm/n* and *lg/w*
> offspring: *sm/n* and *lg/w*
> plus: *sm/w* and *lg/n*

This time recombination has created the two types of particles which were used as parents in the previous experiment.

Now we begin to understand why in the first experiment of this series, where a normal particle and one mutant were used as parents, only these same two types were produced as offspring. It is because in that case no other combinations of characters were possible:

> parents: *sm/n* and *sm/w*
> offspring: *sm/n* and *sm/w*

—and that is all. Consequently this experiment could not reveal whether the DNA is actually treated as a unit during reproduction—as seemed to be the case—or not. More recombination experiments, which we will discuss later, will show that DNA can, in fact, be subdivided to an astonishing extent.

Virus genes

What all this adds up to is that we have now met the gene even in viruses, and in just the same abstract form in which it first presented itself some hundred years ago in higher organisms. Genes were then—and still are—defined as independent units in the hereditary substance of an individual. All together the genes determine the pattern of characteristics, both actual and potential, of the individual. Not all the genes in the hereditary substance of a certain organism will necessarily express themselves in that organism—in part this depends on the environment—but, if conditions are favorable, they *can* express themselves in that organism or its descendants. Fortunately the genes do express themselves in our example; therefore our symbols, which really stand for observable characteristics of the virus, can also be used for the genes which are responsible for the characteristics.

As independent units in the hereditary substance, genes are exchangeable. Gene exchange takes place in every type of sexual reproduction; in fact the term "sexual reproduction" as used in biology is any union, whether or not it involves male and female, which results in a recombination of genes. In this way nature creates new types without having to wait for the rare and unpredictable occurrence of mutation. For this prosaic purpose nature uses "love" in its varied biological forms. We note that, in this sense, even viruses "make love"; we have just been watching them produce recombinations of four different genes.

You will remember that we designated the normal type of phage with the symbols *sm/n*. The symbol *sm* indicates one gene in the hereditary substance and the symbol *n* another. At one time a mutation in a representative of the normal type had led to a new type designated by the symbols *sm/w*. The mutation involved exclusively the gene *n*, which changed to *w*, but not the gene *sm*, which remained unchanged. On another occasion an independent mutation produced the type *lg/n;* here the mutation involved exclusively the gene *sm*, which was changed to *lg*. This leads us to another conclusion about genes which characterizes them as independent units: they mutate independently. A gene which has arisen by mutation from another is called its "allele." Thus in our example *sm* and *lg* are alleles and so are *n* and *w*.

The recombination experiments we have described yielded only the four types, *sm/n, sm/w, lg/n,* and *lg/w;* there were no particles which seemed to contain two alleles of the same gene simultaneously (for example *lg* in addition to *sm,* or *w* in addition to *n*). There are certain exceptions to this rule, but generally it can be assumed that phage particles possess only one specimen of each gene in one or another allele form.

Experimental tricks

Before we return from the abstract gene to the actual structure of DNA encompassing the genes, we had better answer some questions regarding the technical part of re-combination experiments. How is it actually possible to find out what particle types were produced by a partic-ular doubly infected cell? Nothing could be simpler. Enough phages of type *sm/w* as well as type *lg/n* are added to a bacterial suspension so that each cell will, in all probability, get at least one particle of each type. The suspension of doubly infected cells is then diluted with nutrient solution to the point at which a drop of solution contains at most one cell. A large number of single drops are distributed in an equal number of test tubes. Then one awaits the end of the latent period when the cells have burst and scattered their phage yield into the surround-ings, in other words, into the drop in which each cell was suspended. The contents of the test tubes are now distrib-uted, each on a test plate; the number of plaques per plate indicates how many particles were produced by each cell.

How can one tell the types of particles apart, however? If it were only a question of plaque size, there would be no problem; one would simply count the number of big and small plaques per plate. Unfortunately small plaques may derive from type *sm/n* as well as from type *sm/w,* and large plaques from type *lg/n* or *lg/w.* Is it necessary now to take phages from every single plaque and test them on new plates to determine their host range?

Luckily there is a clever short-cut. All four types of phages can be distinguished on one and the same plate if the bacterial lawn is composed of not just one sort of bac-teria but a mixture of two sorts. Half of the bacteria forming the lawn can be infected by all the phage types, whereas the other half are only susceptible to phages containing the gene *w* for "wide host range." Such *w* particles will destroy all bacterial cells and thus make a clear plaque wherever they fall on the mixed lawn. On the other hand, phage particles with the allele *n* for "narrow host range" will only be able to destroy half of the cells in any one spot on the mixed lawn; they will have to leave the other bacteria, which are taboo for them, and the result will be a turbid plaque. The size of the plaque depends, of course, on whether the other gene involved is *sm* or its allele *lg*. Thus four different sorts of plaques are produced, and each can be attributed to one of the four phage types which resulted from the mixture experiment:

sm/w: small clear plaque (parental)
lg/n: large turbid plaque (parental)
sm/n: small turbid plaque (recombinant, "normal")
lg/w: large clear plaque (recombinant, "double mutant")

Figure 27 shows a small section of a test plate where one representative of each of the four phage types happened to settle and produce the appropriate plaque type.

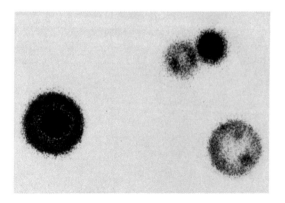

FIG. 27. Four different plaque types from a phage cross. Left bottom: large, clear (type *lg/w*). Right bottom: large, turbid (type *lg/n*). Left top: small, turbid (type *sm/n*). Right top: small, clear (type *sm/w*). (M. Delbrück, *Viruses 1950.* Pasadena, Calif., 1950.)

Gene mapping

Once recombination had been discovered among phages, phage genetics rapidly became a very specialized science because experience gained from years of genetic work with higher organisms could at once be applied. The special interest in phage genetics is that it permits a subdivision of the hereditary substance par excellence, DNA, into functional units. As more and more phage mutants were found and isolated, and used together in recombination experiments, certain general laws began to emerge.

The frequencies of recombinants from crossing experiments turned out to be particularly significant. For instance, a mixed infection with particle types a/c' and a'/c produced about 10 per cent recombinants (a/c and a'/c'); a mixed infection with a/b' and a'/b produced about 3 per cent recombinants (a/b and a'/b'); and a mixed infection with b/c' and b'/c produced about 7 per cent recombinants (b/c and b'/c'). It is to be noted that $3 + 7 = 10$. Is this meaningful or pure coincidence? A large number of further such experiments gave similar results: in any group of three genes and their alleles which were crossed in this way, the largest recombination frequency, expressed as a percentage, was always found to be the sum of the two smaller frequencies. This type of result can be graphically expressed in terms of distance on a line:

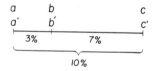

The distance between each pair of alleles is made proportional to the recombination frequency between them. By drawing more and more genes into the experiment and having the diagrams overlap it becomes possible to map all the known genes of a phage particle with respect to their relative recombination frequency. Such a map (for phage T_4) then looks like this:

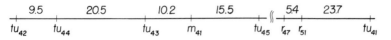

Exchange mechanism

This kind of map is so nice and straightforward that one wonders whether it is not more than just a diagrammatic way of writing recombination frequencies. Doesn't it perhaps indicate the *actual* position of the genes on the DNA strand which somehow must hold them?

This seems indeed to be the case. Diagrams for recombination frequencies were first used in genetic work with higher organisms, where it soon became clear that the genes are contained in linear structures, the chromosomes. Here recombination can even be observed under the microscope, as it takes place. What happens is that two chromosomes simply exchange a section containing the genes which are to be recombined. Here are the two chromosomes:

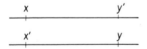

They meet, and one lies crosswise over the other. At the crossing point the two strands break, and each heals with the "wrong" end. When the strands separate again, a gene exchange has taken place.

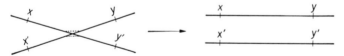

Where the crossing point will be is a matter of chance. Consequently the further apart any two genes are on the strand, the greater the probability of a crossover occurring between them; conversely, the closer together two genes are, the smaller the chance of a crossover between them. In other words, two distant genes will be relatively more frequently recombined than two nearby genes. Thus recombination frequency is, in fact, a measure of the distance between two genes, and the diagrams have in this sense a real relation to the structure of the chromosomes.

How does the recombination mechanism as observed among higher organisms relate to phages? Phages have no visible chromosomes—a chromosome is a giant in comparison to a phage particle—but their hereditary substance, DNA, is a threadlike structure too, lending itself equally well, it seems, to a linear arrangement of genes. One might imagine that, in a mixed infection with two phage types, pieces are exchanged between the entering DNA helices which carry different alleles in a way quite similar to the chromosome mechanism. This conception again underlines the importance of DNA as *the* genetic substance. Chromosomes are complex structures containing many chemical components, including also DNA, so that it is difficult to get at the roots of the matter with them. The genetic material of phages, though it is merely the chemical compound DNA, still shows all the characteristic phenomena of chromosome genetics: divisibility into independent, exchangeable, mutable, functional units which all are lined up in a definite order.

No sooner do we seem to be out of the woods than we run into the thicket. It may appear fairly easy to imagine an exchange of pieces among chromosomes, since these are composed of a large number of segments which are sometimes even visible. Quite possibly the segments do not adhere too tightly, so that breaking and rejoining of pieces can readily occur. On the other hand, DNA helices are held together along their entire length by forces (valences) of the same strength. No chemical reasons exist for assuming any weak spots where the structure might easily break. Such weak spots would have to exist all along the DNA strand if the exchange of pieces were to take place in the same way as between chromosomes.

There might be a thoroughly different mechanism for gene exchange among phages, and further experimental results seem to bear this out. Let us take another look at the diagram of chromosome crossover on p. 125. We note that here each act of recombination must necessarily produce both recombinants. This is in agreement with results of genetic experiments among chromosome-containing organisms. With phages this is not so, however. Only if the particle yield of a great many mixed-infected bacterial cells is counted will the two recombinants make up the same percentage of the total. But if the particle yield of single cells is counted, the two reciprocal types of recombinants do not occur with the same frequency. One cell yields mainly one of the recombinants, whereas the other is hardly represented at all, and with another cell it may be just the opposite. The equal numbers obtained from adding many single yields are thus a purely statistical effect, of little significance to our problem concerning the mechanism of gene exchange as it operates in the individual mixed-infected cell. It begins to look as if this mechanism for DNA helices were in no way comparable to the chromosome mechanism.

Here is another thought, however. Perhaps the unequal recombinant yield from single cells can be explained as a secondary effect. For this we have to fall back upon the DNA pool. You will remember that in this pool there are always some 40–80 DNA helices busily duplicating themselves. While they are supposedly doing this, they would also have plenty of opportunity for sexual promiscuity, that is, the exchange of parts. This they may accomplish in just the same way as chromosomes do, and each act of recombination would then produce two reciprocal recombinants. Since finished helices are taken from the pool at random, however, there is no guarantee that the same number of both recombinant strands will be incorporated into complete phage particles. Of course, the genetic classification technique records only finished phage particles and not such genetic raw material as is still in the pool when the cell bursts. Nevertheless this interpretation is not really convincing, because the discrepancy in the recombinant yield is frequently much greater than would be expected on the basis of random selection. Almost certainly the mechanism of gene exchange between DNA helices is, after all, basically different from the chromosome mechanism.

Conclusions

Phage genetics, as we have noted, is a very large and specialized field in which we do not want to get lost. The purpose of this chapter has been to acquaint the reader with another approach to the general question: How does the structure of nucleic acid relate to its function? In Chapter IV we discussed chemical and physical experiments which seek to first determine the structure and then see what functions such a structure would be capable of. Genetic experiments, on the other hand, record functions and then speculate about the structures which are responsible for these functions. As in the building of a tunnel, the Mountain of the Unknown is being bored from two sides. Already it seems as if one party can hear the drilling of the other, which means that they are moving towards the same point. Soon, perhaps, they will meet.

If we incorporate the facts we learned from phage genetics into our general picture of phage viruses, we arrive at the following: All the genetic information on how to make new phage is carried by the chemical substance DNA contained in every single phage particle. Assuming that all this DNA is in the form of just one giant threadlike molecule, we may think of this molecule as one long "sentence" describing everything involved. The "words" in that sentence are then represented by certain well-defined subsections of the thread. These are the genes, each of which has its definite position in the sentence, i.e., along the thread. Under certain conditions, a gene can be traded for another fairly similar one (allele) which takes its place. This represents a structural change for the nucleic acid molecule and a corresponding change in the "meaning" of the sentence. Such a change can be genetically (but not yet chemically) defined. Virus particles receiving the changed information will have, and pass on, a changed character (recombinants).

As words in a sentence, the genes, in turn, consist of "letters." Four symbols, in the form of four different nucleotides, are available for the construction of letters. Since certainly more than just four letters are required for expressing all that is necessary, groups of nucleotides in specific sequence must be used to build the many necessary letters.

Finally there must be something which separates the nucleotide letters as well as the gene words from each other, otherwise the information would be quite unintelligible. The Morse code, which we have used as an analogy, likewise really employs not two but three signs, namely dot, dash, and pause. A completely continuous series of dots and dashes, without a pause after each group of signs, would be unintelligible even to the most skilled telegraph operator.

How such spaces are indicated in the nucleic acid code is not known. However, on the basis of certain very sensitive recombination experiments with phages it can be estimated how many nucleotides make up the smallest unit—presumably a letter—in this system of writing. Less than a dozen nucleotides is the estimate for this, whereas the entire information for making a phage particle requires 200,000 nucleotides (nucleotide pairs, really, if the double-helix structure is taken into account).

Many a reader will have had an inkling meanwhile that the concepts of phage genetics must have a strong bearing on the thorny problem of nucleic acid reproduction.

It can indeed be shown that gene recombination already takes place during the eclipse, that is, during the period when the cell does not yet contain any complete virus particles. It is definitely known that, once completed, virus particles remain in the cell quite passively and thus do not engage in any more exchange of genetic material. Gene recombination must consequently occur in the same place where copies of the nucleic acid are being made.

If the place for DNA reduplication is the DNA pool, this would have to be the place for gene exchange also. Indeed a mathematical theory has been evolved which explains quantitative recombination effects by regarding the contents of the pool as a population of DNA helices constantly duplicating themselves and constantly exchanging genes with one another. This is a very pleasing theory as it seems to unite two independent groups of experimental data under one hat. The wild confusion in the spaghetti heap is, of course, not reduced if we must now imagine each of the 40–80 DNA strands not only busily duplicating itself, but also ready at any moment to start an affair with its neighbor. It becomes even more difficult to conceive of a mechanism which manages to fish temporarily unengaged helices out of the pool in order to make them into complete virus particles. Yet, whatever the mechanism is, it is very efficient because sometimes as many as thirty new particles are assembled each minute.

Noninheritable changes (modifications)

We must keep in mind that bacteriophages are the only viruses with which clear-cut genetic experiments have so far been possible. Plant viruses are quite hopeless in this respect so that it is not even known whether their nucleic acid is functionally divisible (contains several genes) or not. Apparent recombination effects have been observed after mixed infection with animal viruses, but here the interpretation is a bit questionable. Why this is so can again best be illustrated with phages. Sometimes strange accidents happen in a mixed infection: the cell may pack a new DNA helix of a certain genetic constitution into the "wrong" coat. A mixed infection with particles of different host range, for instance, produces an occasional virus particle with a make-up permitting it to infect cell types it really shouldn't. If it does it will produce nothing but offspring for which that same cell type is taboo. The parent got in once because it was wearing someone else's coat; its DNA then ordered the cell to make particles according to its own recipe—that is to say, with a protein which does *not* fit the receptor substances of this cell type.

Such findings again underline the fact that it is the nucleic acid alone which determines the characteristics of the new virus generation. Whatever way the protein coat is fashioned, none of its characteristics are inherited. Among phages such nongenetic mixing effects are easy to spot, but, for technical reasons, this is not so easy among animal viruses. Therefore, even if a mixed infection of animal viruses seems to produce "recombinants," the observed effects may be due to a nongenetic mixing of parental characteristics. To prove that a genuine gene exchange has taken place it is necessary to show that a particle with mixed characters consistently produces offspring with the same combination of characters.

We mentioned once before that under certain conditions the cell may contribute more than just labor and unspecific building blocks to virus synthesis. It seems that sometimes the cell imposes some of its own specific DNA, that is to say, some of its genes, on the virus particles it is producing. As a result of such a genetic recombination between cell and virus, new virus types with inheritable characteristics are produced even without a mixed infection. To be sure, the recombination is one-sided in this case; it is evident that some virus particles got something from the cell, but what the cell received in exchange from the virus remains unknown; it made virus and had to die before it could reveal anything of its new genetic constitution.

The cell may also make nongenetic contributions to virus synthesis. For instance, a certain phage type may, with a change of host cell, suddenly show changes in practically 100 per cent of its offspring. Return them to the original host type and everything is as it used to be; the new characters seem to be blown away, and can thus not have been genetically fixed. It is said that the new host cell has had a modifying influence, and one speaks of viruses with such reversible character changes as having experienced "virus modifications." Modifications of this sort are also known among higher organisms; they are always caused by certain environmental influences and disappear when the specific influences are removed.

Masked virus

So far we have always maintained that the virus-infected cell is doomed to an early death. Cases are known, however, where cell and virus have joined hands in a bond for life—a precarious sort of bond, to be sure.

Some phage types seem not to do the host cell any harm. The phage is adsorbed and it also injects its DNA into the cell, but the cell doesn't seem to care; it continues to divide, producing numerous apparently normal and healthy daughter cells. In reality each of these descendants carries the devil inside. Expose such a cell to unfavorable conditions, and suddenly all hell breaks loose. As though it had just been attacked by virulent phages—which, of course, is not the case at all—its assembly lines suddenly switch over and make phage particles until the cell bursts. The phages which emerge are always of the same type as that particle which seemed to have shot its bolt in vain many cell generations earlier. How is all this to be explained?

Obviously the DNA from the original phage particle had been incapable of taking complete command over the cell it infected, which continued peaceably in its own way. And so did its daughter cells. The infected mother cell's DNA maintained the upper hand and everything was done in accordance with its directions. The invading virus DNA was not destroyed, however. It managed somehow to settle in, and even got itself copied every time the cell DNA was copied. In this way each descendant of the infected mother cell received, along with its proper inheritance, a recipe for making a certain type of virus. These recipes in the cells remained unused so long as all went well. But as soon as conditions became unfavorable to the cells, the precarious balance was upset and the virus recipe took over.

About this complex phenomenon, known as "lysogeny," a whole book could be written. We have just barely touched on one aspect of the subject which emphasizes once again the central role of nucleic acid as a storage substance for genetic information. A lysogenic cell—that is to say, a latently infected cell—absolutely does not contain a single complete virus particle so long as all is going well; not a trace of virus-specific protein can be found. Nevertheless, a recipe for the manufacture of a specific virus type is passed on from one cell generation to the next. The recipe must be contained in something other than a complete virus particle, presumably a nucleic acid molecule which has worked itself into the genetic apparatus of the cell. Here, for the time being, the virus nucleic acid performs only one of its two main functions—it sees to its own reproduction. The second major function of nucleic acid—to implement its commands—is apparently not necessarily coupled with the first. It seems that this second function can skip any number of generations. Actually it is not clear whether the function switches off completely, or whether attempts by the virus nucleic acid to assert itself are continuously suppressed or reversed by the healthy lysogenic cell.

"Masked" virus occurs among higher organisms too,

and makes certain virus diseases very baffling. Take, for instance, the case of swine influenza. The virus for this disease is taken in by a lung worm which parasitizes the pig. The lung worm passes the virus into its eggs which find their way out through the intestinal canal of the pig. Once outside, the eggs are eaten by an earthworm. Inside the earthworm, the lung worm larvae emerge, go through certain stages of development, and then they wait until the earthworm is eaten by a pig. After some further developmental steps, they get back into the pig lung where they become mature lung worms. However, there is no influenza yet for the pig containing the lung worms with latent virus. A further stimulus must be added in the form of an infection of the pig by a normally harmless bacillus, and furthermore all this must not be during May, June, July, or August. If all these conditions are fulfilled, influenza suddenly breaks out. The virus is now fully infectious and can also be directly transferred from pig to pig. In the intermediate hosts—lung worm and earthworm—no active virus could ever be found. How the masking of the virus is accomplished in this case is not known, and, fascinating though it all is, the reader will agree that lysogenic bacteria are more convenient for this type of study.

We note that, unlike most viruses, whose host range is restricted to a small number of related cell types, the swine influenza virus is taken in by several completely different hosts. Whether reproduction of the virus takes place only in the pig, or in the worm hosts too, is not known. There are cases, however, where it is quite certain that the same virus can multiply in organisms as different as a plant and an insect. Plant viruses are transmitted by insects which take up the virus along with the sap of a diseased plant and transfuse it to other plants. Usually the infectiousness of such insects is soon lost if they are kept away from infected plants. In certain cases, however, the insects remain infectious throughout twenty generations and more, even though they never again come in contact with infectious plants. The virus must be passed on to each succeeding generation with the eggs, and it must also have multiplied in the insects, or else it would have been diluted out long before the twentieth generation. It can also be shown directly that the virus multiplies in a single artificially infected insect. Contrary to the plants, the insects usually show no disease symptoms.

That a virus should be able to multiply in such different host organisms is not so utterly surprising at first sight, since we recall that host specificity is often determined merely by specific receptor-substances (which do not exist in plants). Just the same, all plant viruses are not infectious for all plants. In the above example not only plant but also insect cells have to be infected by the virus, and thus receptor substances might after all be involved during the insect phase of the reproductive cycle.

VI. *The Heart of the Matter*

Are there really autocatalytic reproductive systems?

The central importance of DNA in the hereditary mechanism of phages and also of cells has been emphasized again and again. It must be obvious, therefore, how nice it would be if one could be sure that DNA reproduces itself by itself and thus finally closes the reproductive cycle.

Originally an even more complex biological unit than DNA—the whole virus particle—was thought to be capable of autocatalytic reproduction. This idea had to be given up as soon as it was found that the particle does not remain a unit during reproduction. Investigators were then forced back to the DNA, for what could not be true for the whole particle might still be true for a part. Yet instinct tells us that there must be an end somewhere to the splitting up of a whole which is to be reproduced.

Maybe so, but the end doesn't have to be where one would like to see it. There is no indisputable evidence against the possibility that, after the virus particle is split up during infection, its DNA is further dismembered by the cell, and thus loses its structural identity. What if the cell can only "read" the DNA strands by treating them as chemical agents and involving them in reactions which change their structure? After all, the only important thing is that the *information* be retained. The erstwhile material carrier can change; having delivered the information, it has done its duty, and its remains may be as unimportant as the empty protein coat of the phage particle, which was left hanging outside the cell wall right at the beginning of infection. Once a recipe has been learned by heart, the paper on which it was written can be thrown away.

Experiments described so far seem to fit the conception of a nucleic acid strand which is self-reproducing and remains structurally intact. Nevertheless, it is also possible that the DNA strand from the infecting particle sacrifices its structural identity, just as the whole particle did, in order to "prime the pumps" in a more complicated manner and get the cell to set up machinery making new virus particles, DNA and all. One could even imagine—and certain findings seem to suggest this—that the first few newly produced DNA strands are "read" by the cell in the same way, that is, immediately broken down again, until with several sets of machinery the production really gets rolling. Once this has been accomplished, the newly made strands could then begin to accumulate and await in complete inertia the packaging into their protein coats. What peace in this kind of DNA pool as compared with the heap of madly mating and reduplicating DNA helices!

Uncertain fate of the infecting virus nucleic acid

Some consequences of the alternative possibilities can be experimentally tested. If the two halves of the infecting DNA double helix remain intact in the cell when the structure starts a pool of daughter helices all on its own, as the proposed autocatalytic reproductive mechanism would require, then these two old strands should finally wind up again in protein coats and reappear in exactly two particles of the new generation of phages. At any rate, allowing for complications (recombination by breaks, etc.), the total matter of the infecting DNA should be found among the DNA of the new phage particles. If, on the other hand, the infecting DNA strand immediately transfers its information to other structures in the cell, during which process it is destroyed and made useless, then none of its atoms ought to reappear in the new phage generation.

It should be possible to resolve this question by using radioactive atoms as tracers. If a bacterial culture is infected with phage particles whose DNA has been marked with radioactive atoms it can be determined how much of this radioactive material reappears in the new phage generation.

Alas, the result of such experiments is, of all things, this: approximately half of the original DNA is recovered, and the other half not! Nature is leading the ingenious experimenter by the nose. Unhappy man, the best he can do now is to try and explain the result according to his preference. He may try to save the autocatalytic method by explaining away the missing 50 per cent as unimportant, or, on the other hand, he may claim that the recovered 50 per cent is unimportant and got into the new phage particles accidentally.

In fact, the situation is even more involved, as more experiments along these lines have shown. We will have to content ourselves with discussing a little further the outcome of the basic experiment described above. The convinced proponent of autocatalytic DNA reproduction, who sets up the recovered 50 per cent as the only significant portion of the infecting DNA, runs into all kinds of difficulties. Logically he must assert that this half of the original strand is still capable of self-reproduction and also still contains all the genetic information. This conception, however, endangers the main argument for the autocatalytic method, the DNA model. What would the difference be between self-reproducible and nonreproducible DNA?

The believer in an indirect reproductive method cannot feel very happy with the experimental result either, though the unexpectedly recovered 50 per cent can be explained easily enough. If the DNA, on delivering its information, is broken down, then the resulting pieces could be used again as unspecific building material to make new specific virus DNA. The cell is not dependent on this minor supply, of course; its assembly lines can turn out infinitely more DNA precursor material, but since the breakdown pieces are around, they might as well be used. Yet what about the other 50 per cent? Perhaps they are chemically useless DNA fragments, or else this portion of the original DNA is needed for specific jobs, for instance in the maturation machinery for tailoring coats, or some other apparatus of virus reproduction which the cell lacks in the beginning.

Protein as the middleman?

We already know that proteins, in the form of enzymes, play an important middleman role whenever complex chemical transformations have to be accomplished in the cell. Thus, in the event of indirect DNA replication, protein could also take over the directions from the DNA and carry them out. This would mean that some special proteins would have to be constructed immediately following infection, and before any new virus DNA can be produced.

The following experiment seems to support this idea: A phage-infected cell actually makes a considerable amount of protein which has nothing to do with later protein coats for new phage particles. If a freshly infected bacterial cell is prevented from synthesizing any protein (this can be done with certain chemical tricks), then no virus DNA is synthesized either. If the blockade is then removed, first protein synthesis, and then also DNA synthesis is resumed. Having once been set in motion, however, DNA synthesis cannot be stopped by later blocking of protein synthesis.

Results of another type of experiment equally support the idea that protein acts as middleman in the copying process of DNA. By replacing a great deal of the normal phosphorus atoms of the DNA in phage particles by radioactive phosphorus, one makes a preparation of "hot" phage. Hot phage rapidly commit suicide, that is, lose their ability to multiply, because the decay of the built-in radioactive phosphorus atoms disrupts the DNA structure, thereby wiping out the genetic information carried by it. Cells are infected with these hot phage before they can commit suicide, and the multiplication process is left running for just a few minutes. It is then interrupted until all hot phage DNA within the cell must be destroyed. Will the cells, when brought back to metabolic activity, now be able to finish their job of making new phage? Yes, they will! In the short interval between infection and interruption of the phage multiplication, the genetic information of the phage must have been taken from the endangered DNA and stored in some other safe structure. It doesn't matter now whether the original virus DNA, as well as any newly produced virus DNA, disintegrates —the cell does not lose the ability to make more virus. All recipes are torn, but the cell has learned her lesson by heart. Protein does not contain any phosphorus and is thus safe from radioactive disintegration. It is therefore the worthiest candidate for any guesses on which structure might have stored the information.

In addition to these results as arguments for an indirect reproductive system, we must consider the fact that many viruses have ribonucleic acid (RNA) instead of DNA as the carrier of genetic information. It is now quite certain, however, that RNA is not constructed on the principle of paired bases. Therefore the model for autocatalytic reproduction based on the DNA double helix cannot apply to RNA. Is it likely that nature has evolved two completely different self-replicating systems with two chemically so closely related materials? This close relation

makes both DNA and RNA suitable for coding by nucleotide sequences, which may eventually turn out to be of
much greater importance than any notion of a structure
that should reproduce autocatalytically.

It is hard to predict what detours and complications an
indirect reproductive system would involve. No doubt one
of the great advantages of the autocatalytic theory, based
on the DNA model, is its straightforwardness. This theory
has led and is still leading to all kinds of interesting experiments, and even if it should some day be proven
wrong, it will have been most useful.

It is really quite a problem even to design experiments
which would track down an indirect reproductive system.
For one thing, there are too many possibilities. Does the
intermediary protein act simply as a stamping machine,
which continuously stamps out copies of the nucleic acid
molecule to which it owes its own existence? Can an individual nucleic acid molecule make only one such stamping machine, or several? Is it possible for two different
stamping machines to work hand in hand and thus produce genetic recombinants? One perhaps begins a copy,
whereas the other one finishes it. Might this possibly explain the unequal frequencies of "reciprocal" recombinants? How is one to devise experiments which will give
a clear-cut answer to even one of these questions?

Goals for further research

On the whole, we must conclude that research in this
field has reached a state where a basic and bold new step
is required: the attempt to remove the nucleic acid reproductive system from the cell and transplant it into the
test tube. If successful, this feat would be comparable to
the first production of a yeast extract which was cell-free
but nevertheless capable of fermentation. Had it been
necessary to study the transformation of sugar into alcohol and carbon dioxide entirely within the cell, then the
various steps in the fermentation process would, no

doubt, still be a mystery. It was the yeast extract which made it possible to take the system apart piece by piece, put it back together again, and test what happened each time. Thus each material which takes part in the process could be isolated and its function determined.

Similarly, if the nucleic acid reproductive system could be extracted from the cell it would be much easier to study. The technical difficulties of transplanting such a system into a test tube are, of course, much greater than they were in connection with the fermentation process, yet certainly not as great as the problem of reconstructing a complete living system from its components. For the present it would be very nice if one could extract from cells something which under the direction of an added trace of genetically specific nucleic acid could make more of the same out of simple building blocks. Of course it would be even nicer if the isolated system could take some given phage nucleic acid and some simple building blocks and make complete phage particles out of these. Even this, as we know, would still be far from a living system.

Perhaps we shall someday see these wishes fulfilled.

VII. *Control of Virus Disease*

During our sojourn in the realm of pure science we seem to have almost forgotten that viruses cause disease which one would like to get rid of. What advice can the scientist give in this practical endeavor? To state it briefly: not much. But, as a result of basic research with viruses, he can at least say why good advice is hard to give, and so can the reader if the previous chapters have succeeded in their aim.

Cure

The crux of the difficulty is this: Viruses can only multiply by means of the chemical assembly lines of cells, whereby these are severely damaged or even destroyed. Thus viruses cause disease because of their manner of reproduction. To make them harmless it would be necessary to prevent them from multiplying, but obviously one cannot use any means for this which would halt the assembly lines. Such means, which of course stop virus production in every infected cell, do exist. But they also kill all the healthy cells in the organism. Remedies which act on the principle of assembly-line blockage, and which have worked wonders with bacterial infections (penicillin,

streptomycin, terramycin, sulfanilamide, etc.), are therefore of no use in combatting virus diseases. Bacterial infections present quite a different situation. Here too the
causal agents must be stopped from multiplying in the infected organism. Bacteria, however, are independent living things; they have chemical assembly lines of their own
which differ in certain particulars from those of the host
cells. Consequently there are chemical substances which
can be used specifically to block the bacterial assembly
lines without affecting those of the host organism.

A straightforward chemical attack on viruses, in so far
as they can be caught outside of the host cell, is also
likely to be dangerous. Virus particles consist of protein
and nucleic acid, two compounds which likewise occur
in every living cell. Chemicals which can destroy nucleic
acid or protein or both certainly exist, but to use them as
"cures" would be like chasing out the Devil with Beelze-
bub. Perhaps in certain cases a chemical might be found
which limits its destructive activity to the fine structure
of a certain protein and leaves all other proteins alone.
The structure of protein includes enough chemical vari-
ants to make this at least conceivable, whereas the much
more uniform fine structure of nucleic acid molecules will
probably never permit such selective attack.

Further research may uncover points in the reproductive cycle of viruses which are unexpectedly vulnerable
to specific therapeutic attack. For example, whereas the
enzymatic apparatus used for virus production is part of
the cell, this is certainly not true of the end product,
which is virus, and thus foreign. It might be possible, by
external action, to induce the infected cell to make a
slightly different end product, for instance inactive virus
particles. In this way, although all cells which are already
infected would be doomed, the further reproduction of
the virus would at least be halted and the infection
checked.

Inactive virus has been obtained according to this principle. Along with the usual nutrients, virus-infected cells are offered an abnormal chemical derivative of one of the four bases which go to make up nucleic acid. The chemical machinery of the cells does not notice the change and the altered base is built into the virus nucleic acid in place of the normal one. This changes the information carried by the nucleic acid of the newly made virus particles and makes it "illegible" to the next host cells, which then cannot reproduce the virus. Incidentally it is interesting to note that the cell thus can make a DNA it would be unable to read. A closer look at this fact will convince the reader that it is most difficult to reconcile this with autocatalytic DNA reproduction.

Laboratory research also turned up the chance discovery that a certain dye stuff seems to prevent the nucleic acid and protein coat from being assembled into complete virus particles. Practically speaking, not much that is useful has so far come out of such theoretically very interesting discoveries. Mostly this is because the effect must be directed with utter specificity towards cells which are already infected. This is difficult to do even in the laboratory, and would be impossible in a patient.

When we try to think up ways to catch free virus particles outside the cells, we recall that some viruses require receptor substances to enter the host cell. Such receptor substances can be extracted and, in so far as the reaction between them and the viruses is irreversible, they make fine inactivating agents. Unfortunately, just those viruses which are of the greatest practical interest—because they are most dangerous to man—are the ones which can free themselves from receptor substances to which they were attached. The receptor substance would have to be chemically treated in such a way that it binds and refuses to be detached again. Attempts in this direction seem to have met with some success, though not as yet of practical importance.

Receptor specificity applies only to some virus types,

but all viruses have a characteristic serological specificity. Virus protein induces warm-blooded animals to make
antibodies which are then found in the blood serum. The
antibodies, also protein, will combine specifically with the
protein that induced them. Thus the virus particles can
be enveloped within the appropriate antibody, and this
usually inactivates them, presumably because they cannot
get rid of the antibody layer. The serum of humans or
animals who have had a certain disease can actually be
used to combat the disease in others. Where adequate
amounts of pure virus are available, considerable quantities of specific antiserum can be obtained by, for instance,
immunizing horses or other large animals with the virus
and then drawing off some of the blood. Animals which
are used for this purpose do not have to get the disease or
even be susceptible to it; the introduction of a foreign
body is alone sufficient to induce the production of the
desired antibodies. This method is not limited to viruses;
it is also used to make diphtheria antiserum and other
antiserums.

Prevention

Serum treatment is expensive and it often is not very,
or not at all, effective, largely because it tends to come too
late. It would be much better if it could be arranged for
the endangered individual already to have the appropriate antibodies in his bloodstream before he becomes
infected with the virus. A preventive injection of antiserum, called passive immunization, is not usually very effective, and repeated injections may be quite dangerous
Luckily, however, nature has provided us all with the ability to make our own antibodies. Of course nobody would
be quite so mad as to purposely infect himself with virus
in order to become immune (on the principle that an end
with horror is better than horror without end). As already
indicated, however, antibody production is possible without disease. Only the protein is needed to induce the de-

sired antibodies, and so long as it is not part of an active virus particle, the protein is not dangerous. Therefore you can have yourself injected with virus particles which have been inactivated so skillfully that the protein has remained, as far as possible, intact. This is not easy to achieve, of course, and consequently certain dangers are inherent in active immunization. Yet with adequately controlled technique, active immunization has many advantages; in the treatment of such dangerous diseases as poliomyelitis and yellow fever it is indispensable because nothing else is known which works nearly so well.

Sometimes even active virus, for example yellow fever virus, is used for immunization purposes. However, it is a weakened virus which can scarcely produce symptoms in man; its virulence has been bred out during many generations of growing in the laboratory on tissue cultures of somewhat uncongenial host cells, such as chicken eggs. During this weakening process the virus retains its serological specificity but loses other characteristics, for instance a predilection for certain cell types which are vital to the human host. This "passage technique" can be successfully applied to a number of different viruses. It involves either modifications or selection of mutants which were present in the original stock and were given their chance to become dominant when unfavorable conditions inhibited the reproduction of the normal type. It has long been known that human-pathogenic viruses can be weakened and made usable as vaccines by passing them through animals (cow pox, rabies); the principle of selection was unconsciously applied here before it was recognized as such.

Active immunization is a preventive measure, and prevention is about the only defense against virus diseases we have at present. Therapy is useful only if it promises to do considerably less harm than good, and for viruses no such therapy has really been developed yet. Since we must depend on prevention rather than cure, therefore, the individual suffering from a rare virus disease, or a relatively harmless one like the common cold, is quite helpless. Prevention, if it is to be effective, must generally be carried out on a large scale; it tends to be costly and may require obligatory measures on the part of the government which are justified only if the disease in question holds great danger to many people. That even simple preventive measures can be very effective if they are thoroughly carried out is illustrated by the nearly complete suppression of yellow fever in populated areas due to the eradication of the mosquito carrier.

Preventive measures are also the weapon of choice against those plant viruses that often are of great economic importance because of their effect on the harvest. Occasionally it has been possible to cure a diseased plant by dipping it into hot water for a short time or letting it grow at supernormal temperatures for a while. Of course this sort of treatment cannot be applied to a field of potatoes or beets or sugar cane, but it might be of some practical importance in the production of virus-free seedlings.

Chemicals like insecticides, which could be dusted over a whole field to cure plants of virus diseases, would be a big business, but they don't exist yet and maybe never will.

Breeding

A measure which cannot be applied to humans but which is of considerable importance with plants and sometimes with animals is the breeding of virus-resistant races. Several degrees of virus-resistance can be distinguished. The ideal would be complete immunity, in which the virus disease does not even take hold. Also desirable, though less effective, is relative resistance, for instance mild symptoms or quick recovery of the affected organisms. Finally there is a third kind of resistance which should really be called "tolerance." It is very popular in plant-breeding circles; temporarily it produces the desired effect, but potentially it is very dangerous. Virus-tolerant plants are by no means resistant; they simply show no symptoms of disease. They can be crawling with viruses without this having any effect on the harvest yield, but this is just the dangerous aspect of the matter. Soon practically all existing stocks of such plants will be infested with the virus. Because of the enormous danger of infection, more susceptible varieties of the same plant can no longer be grown at all, even though it might be desirable to do so. Furthermore, the huge virus-reservoir which is accumulating in the tolerant plants offers an excellent opportunity for normally rare mutants to occur in greater numbers. Some mutants, as we know, are distinguished by an increased host range; they may suddenly cause epidemics of virus disease among plants which were previously quite unaffected. Other mutants may even become dangerous to the tolerant stock, due to a change in virulence. Thus, in the long run, tolerant races may be more risky than profitable. Incidentally, every type of resistance, even absolute immunity, can, at any time, be broken by a suitable type of virus mutant appearing on the scene all of a sudden. Thus the breeder is engaged in a continuous race against his mutable enemy; never can he rest comfortably on his laurels.

Where a virus is transmitted from plant to plant by insects only, there is, of course, the possibility of directing defensive measures against the insects. Attempts in this direction have not been as successful as in the suppression of yellow fever, however. A better plan in such cases seems to be to try to breed plants which are avoided by the virus-carrying insects.

Where all else fails, the only remedy is ruthless destruction of all visibly diseased or even obviously exposed plants. If this involves trees which take a long time to grow, such as cacaos, it can be a costly procedure which the planter may well be reluctant to carry through.

The animal breeder's scope is more limited than that of

the plant breeder because there are usually fewer domestic animals available which can be examined for resistant individuals. Also it would be an expensive proposition to sacrifice the milk and meat yield of a whole herd of cattle, let us say, by exposing them to hoof-and-mouth disease in the hope of finding a few resistant animals for breeding purposes. Since even successful breeds are always subject to the dangers of virus mutability, the only really successful measures here are destruction of diseased stocks and, where valuable large animals are involved, quarantine and active immunization. Unfortunately, immunization is not proof against virus mutability either. If a mutant with altered serological characters but unchanged pathogenic traits crops up, then the whole immunization program has been in vain.

All in all it would certainly be a great boon if a chemotherapeutic treatment against at least the worst of the virus diseases could some day be found. At the moment, unfortunately, there is not much basis for optimism.

VIII. *What Is Virus and Where Does It Come From?*

We have now touched on everything concerning virus, and some aspects we have discussed in considerable detail. Nevertheless the reader will find it difficult to say in a few words just what a virus is. On the other hand, he will know why this is difficult. A description of the virus particle alone would leave out just the most important characteristics. As soon as these characteristics come into play, however, the virus particle as such ceases to exist! In its place we find a complex chemo-dynamic system where the different components of the particle interact at different times with the most diversified components of a living organism—the host cell. As an end product of all this activity we again find that seemingly innocent and uninteresting structure, the virus particle.

Analogy

Perhaps it is easiest to explain what a virus is by means of an analogy. A large machine factory will represent the cell. Engineers and workers build machines according to plan, and with function and work rhythms carefully coordinated. Raw materials are taken in and converted into machines. These end products are used to replace worn-out models, as reserves, and are also sold (which is merely a special way of tapping sources for the supply of energy and raw material) to feed the workers and keep them functioning (which includes their having children). If such a production system is well balanced it lives forever; its output of machines and new workers is always the same in the same period of time; as a whole and in all its parts it works arithmetically. In the event of overproduction, identical daughter systems, that is, new factories, can be split off. If raw material supplies and markets are steady, the founding of new factories can be repeated rhythmically so that the number of such systems, and consequently also their total output, grows geometrically with time, even though each individual system works arithmetically.

Now suppose that somehow one of these beautifully balanced factories or production cycles is infiltrated by a misfit—a wrong blueprint from the construction department, let us say. Nobody notices. The interloper is swept up into the work cycle, and everything is now done according to its directions. The assembly lines are redirected and produce an (arithmetic) series of lovely new machines which, however, don't function and are also unsalable. The business goes bankrupt, while the nice new machines are left standing around because nobody wants them. In the analogy they represent the virus particles, of course.

We can even spin our tale a little further. A competing firm sees the attractive machines standing idle. Thinking them excellent because it knows nothing of the bankruptcy, it steals one, has it taken apart, carefully copied, and put into production. Soon this firm too goes broke, and so does any other which is similarly taken in.

Mistakes

It is quite possible that viruses first arose, just as in the analogy, because of a mistake. Something went wrong in the central office of some cell during the copying of a production recipe. Such a mistake does not necessarily merely cause an assembly line to be blocked. In addition, the faulty recipe could conceivably become independent by overthrowing the balance of the whole system and causing it to produce an unproportionately large number of copies of itself. It would do the same in any other cell it manages to enter. In this case the erstwhile mistake has become a sort of parasitic molecule, unable, of course, to do anything by itself, but certain of always forcing organized systems blindly to do its bidding whenever it can sneak in.

Runaways

A mistake in copying is not the only way imaginable by which chemical parasites could be created. Possibly a molecular complex which behaves quite sensibly and usefully in the cell where it belongs goes berserk if it happens to get into another type of cell where it doesn't fit. The chance transfer of components of one cell into another can happen in any number of ways. Insects, for instance, constantly carry various cell components (not only viruses) from one plant or animal to another.

Of course it is only recipe-type components which would be capable of assuming virus character. This limits the range of possible virus precursors to nucleic acid-containing structures. Where nucleic acid is involved, the capability to mutate also exists. Thus through the mechanisms of mutation and selection the former cell component can rapidly develop further and further away from its original form, until it becomes impossible to trace back to its birthplace.

This is why we don't know for sure whether viruses

actually arose in either of the ways just described. If they did, then there is no reason why the process should not still be going on, creating new viruses and consequently also new virus diseases. There are some indications that this is indeed happening.

Theories

What about the old idea that viruses are precursors of life? It is to be hoped that no reader of this book will fall for that any more. Cells, with their complex dynamic organization, are the absolutely essential prerequisite for virus propagation, and life must therefore have begun on the cellular level. Even if some spontaneous act of generation had brought a virus particle forth from some sort of primordial slime, that particle would have remained lonely and forgotten forever without the simultaneous presence of living cells.

At the present time attempts are being made to artificially re-create such a primordial slime. In a mixture of simple substances like steam, methane, ammonia, and hydrogen—an atmosphere that may have enveloped the earth some billions of years ago—and under the influence of electric discharge, certain simple organic compounds, for instance amino acids, can arise. This is undoubtedly very interesting, but amino acids are not proteins by a long shot, and even a mixture of somehow spontaneously arisen proteins and nucleic acids does not constitute a self-reproducing cyclical organization. Either those manifold interdependent members of a complete cycle arise or at least gather together spontaneously at one moment and at one tiny spot (which is hard to imagine), or else a mixture of even the most complex molecules remains what it is: a collection of chemical compounds.

The problem of the origin of life is but a special case of the fundamentally and equally unsolved problem of biological evolution as a whole, which is sometimes phrased in the mock-serious question: Which came first, the chicken or the egg? It is safe to say that we don't even have the beginnings of an answer to the question of spontaneous generation, nor are we likely to get it from the study of viruses. The prospects of getting it from pure philosophy are much worse, though.

Viruses help us to solve the riddle of life in other ways, however, such as by allowing us to study the functioning of ready-made living systems at the lowest level. Thanks to viruses this riddle is slowly moving into the class of crossword puzzles: we know the principles on which the puzzle operates, and now all that has to be done is to find the key words and fit them into the scheme. This will still require a lot of work and worry and bright ideas, but it is not impossible.

A hundred years ago the situation was much more confusing. Astrology, magic, vitalism—all kinds of theories seemed possible and found their fanatic supporters. Problems must be ripe for their solution, and before they are, nothing very sensible can be said about them. Occasionally, though, we may review the state of our knowledge in order to see whether it is possible to answer any of the old questions. Admittedly, such self-restraint may be a bit difficult to observe, for who wouldn't prefer having the answers to certain well-known questions in his lifetime.

INDEX

Now available

Ann Arbor Science Library Paperbacks

AAS 501   **THE STARS** by W. Kruse and W. Dieckvoss

AAS 502   **THE ANTS** by Wilhelm Goetsch

AAS 503   **THE SENSES** by Wolfgang von Buddenbrock

AAS 504   **LIGHT: VISIBLE AND INVISIBLE** by Eduard Ruechardt

AAS 505   **THE BIRDS** by Oskar and Katharina Heinroth

AAS 506   **EBB AND FLOW: The Tides of Earth, Air, and Water** by Albert Defant

AAS 507   **ANIMAL CAMOUFLAGE** by Adolf Portmann

AAS 508   **PLANET EARTH** by Karl Stumpff

AAS 509   **VIRUS** by Wolfhard Weidel

AAS 510   **THE SUN** by Karl Kiepenheuer

and other titles to follow

The University of Michigan Press